THE WOMAN'S BOOK OF SLEEP

A Complete Resource Guide

AMY R. WOLFSON, PH.D.

FOREWORD BY KATHRYN A. LEE, R.N., PH.D.

NEW HARBINGER PUBLICATIONS, INC.

Distributed in Canada by Raincoast Books

Copyright © 2001 by Amy Wolfson
                New Harbinger Publications, Inc.
                5674 Shattuck Avenue
                Oakland, CA 94609

Cover image: La Dormeuse by Tamara de Lempicka, © 2001 Artists Rights Society (ARS), New York/ADAGP, Paris
Cover design by Salmon Studios
Edited by Karen O'Donnell Stein
Text design by Tracy Marie Carlson

Library of Congress Card Catalog Number: 01-132308

ISBN-10 1-57224-249-3
ISBN-13 978-1-57224-249-4

All Rights Reserved

Printed in the United States of America

New Harbinger Publications' Web site address: www.newharbinger.com

09   08   07

10   9   8   7   6   5   4   3   2

In memory
of my mother and best friend,
Judith P. Wolfson,
who taught me wonderful sleep habits
years before I ever became a psychologist and sleep researcher.

Contents

Foreword

As I buckled my seat belt and prepared for the five-hour flight back home to San Francisco from Washington, D.C., I made sure that I had easy access to Dr. Wolfson's final draft of this book and my new John Grisham novel. It was only 4:30 A.M. in San Francisco when I left Dulles airport at 7:30 A.M., and I had just completed an intense two days of work in Washington with little sleep. My plan was to take a nap after reading a few chapters from this book and get started on the novel. Well, I never made it to my nap or the novel! I read the entire set of manuscript pages for Dr. Wolfson's book and started to write this foreword before I landed back in San Francisco.

How she had time to write such a thorough book and include such up-to-date information, with her busy teaching and research schedule, is a mystery to me. But it is no mystery that Dr. Wolfson is a dedicated scientist and expert on this topic. She says she wrote this book for women. However, I have to respectfully disagree. What struck me most about this book, its contents, and the way in which it is written, is that it is definitely *not* just for women. Although women do suffer from sleep problems more often than men, men would also benefit greatly from the information contained in this book—not just to understand their mothers, wives, or daughters, but to understand their own personal sleep-related health.

Written in an engaging style, this book takes us through the relevant physiology we need in order to understand the sleep issues within each chapter as well as the "Sleep-Smart Strategies" Dr. Wolfson presents at the conclusion of each chapter. We learn through reading this book that Dr. Wolfson is not only a busy professional herself, but also a wife and a mother. Her examples, from her own personal life as well as from diverse women who participated in her research studies, make the content real and relevant to today's busy working women as we experience modern societal pressures on a daily basis.

Dr. Wolfson has tackled the complexities of female physiology related to sleep that most sleep researchers have managed to avoid since research first began in sleep laboratories in the early 1950s. Not only is the physiology presented in an easy-to-understand format—she obviously took great pains to make it sound so simple and straightforward—yet so accurate and detailed. She presents the complex physiology of women's health, hormones, and cycles in a way that should be read by all adults, whether or not one they have a problem with sleep.

Sleep—what is normal and healthy, or what is abnormal and problematic—is a relatively new area of scientific inquiry. As Dr. Wolfson explains, we are learning a great deal more about the functions and dysfunctions of sleep every day. But we still know very little about sleep problems women experience at key times in their lives, like pregnancy and menopause. My particular opinion is that we can learn even more when we follow Dr. Wolfson's example and include women as subjects in sleep research studies, rather than ignore them because of the complexities of their hormonal functions. For instance, Dr. Wolfson discusses the important relationship between body temperature fluctuations and sleep patterns. Yet most of this knowledge comes from manipulating the temperature of male subjects in a laboratory setting. Could there be a better natural experiment than to study women, who have temperatures that fluctuate every month with ovulation, temperatures that increase during pregnancy, and temperatures that fluctuate hourly during menopausal hot flashes? A researcher would not have to perform complex manipulations of the subject's temperature if only the research subject were a woman—just wait a few minutes or days, and it will change without drugs, blankets, or hot tubs!

I thoroughly enjoyed reading this book, and actually was surprised that I remained awake for the entire flight, particularly since the content in these ten chapters is already familiar to me, I was suffering from jet lag, and I had had little sleep during the previous week. If you are planning to read this book all in one sitting, as I did, it is possible to do just that. But if you are planning to sit down to read and digest one chapter at a time, as Dr. Wolfson recommends, you will still benefit even more from the new knowledge you gain at each sitting. If you are planning to read this at night to help you fall asleep, I can tell you that it probably won't happen. The information is presented in a way that is just too engaging, and I didn't sleep a wink, even in my sleep-deprived state on the airplane.

Dr. Wolfson's approach—that you can best help yourself sleep better when you understand your own unique sleep needs and the physiological basis behind them—is one that women can best relate to. You will need to read the important information, and the Sleep-Smart Strategies in the pages that follow, in order to learn how best to do that for your own particular sleep issue, or to help your family members and friends. Just as on airplanes you are advised to apply the oxygen mask to yourself first, then to your child, you can apply the information in this book to yourself, and then to others around you.

Most adults, but particularly women, will find they can relate to many of the situations presented by Dr. Wolfson and the many women she has studied over the years. I know I did. Like myself, you will want to keep this book handy on your bookshelf, since the resources Dr. Wolfson provides in the back will be helpful to you long after you finish reading this book. Enjoy the book, and pleasant dreams!

Kathryn A. Lee, R.N., Ph.D., F.A.A.N. (Fellow in the American Academy of Nursing)
Professor, Family Health Care Nursing
Director, Perinatal Nursing Master's Program
James and Marjorie Livingston Chair in Nursing

Acknowledgments

I have dedicated this book to the memory of my mother, Judith P. Wolfson, who died at the young age of sixty-two, just three years ago. In addition, I dedicate this book to the memory of my colleague Dr. Helen Bearpark. Shortly before Helen died she signed a contract with editors at New Harbinger to write a book on women's sleep. Several years later, New Harbinger approached me to write a book on women's sleep, not knowing that I had known and admired Helen Bearpark. In fact, just before she died, she and I talked over coffee at the College of the Holy Cross, where I teach, regarding some of the ways that she and I could begin to collaborate on research on women's sleep-wake patterns. Knowing that Helen never had a chance to write her book on women's sleep has motivated and inspired me throughout this past year to create an informative, clear, and helpful book on women's sleep over the lifespan that would be beneficial to women and their health-care providers.

I would like to publicly acknowledge a few significant mentors over the years. First, I would like to thank my graduate-school professors, Dr. Patricia Lacks and Dr. Amy Bertelson, who turned me on to sleep research while I was a doctoral student at Washington University in St. Louis. Second, I am forever grateful to Dr. Mary Carskadon and her colleague Dr. Christine Acebo of the E. P. Bradley Hospital Sleep Laboratory, Brown University Medical School, for their ongoing friendship, expertise, guidance, and inspiration regarding sleep research. Third, I'd like to thank Dr. Ursula Anwer, neurologist at UMASS Memorial Sleep Disorders Center, for her collaboration on our study of women's sleep and mood from the last trimester of pregnancy through twelve months postpartum.

I owe an enormous debt to four very special young women who, as Holy Cross undergraduates, worked as my research assistants for this book: Tatum Charron, Lisa Goncalvez, Melanie

Graham, and Christina Rossi. Without these four dedicated, bright, and hardworking young women, this book would not have been possible. They kept me on schedule, accepted my absentmindedness, and cheered me on throughout the process. Specifically, Tatum Charron assisted with the glossary and citations, Christina Rossi worked diligently on the resources and appendixes, Melanie Graham assisted with the resources, and Lisa Goncalvez helped develop the sleep-wake diary and coordinate one of my earlier studies on women's sleep.

A number of my earlier research assistants also deserve recognition. Much of the data discussed in chapter 6 on working women's sleep-wake patterns would not have been collected if it were not for the help of four Holy Cross graduates, Katherine Harrison, Holly Khachadoorian, Melissa Flynn, and Andrea Flynn. My research on women's sleep from the last trimester of pregnancy through twelve months postpartum came out of a true collaboration with one of my honor students, Jennifer Bassett, and my colleague, Dr. Ursula Anwer. The three of us worked together on the design and implementation of this study, which is referred to in chapter 4. In addition, I wholeheartedly thank my research assistants for their tireless work on this particular study: Sarah Barnes, Christina Cirrone, Stephanie Crowley, Alicia Hoag, Victoria Marcelino, Kathleen McGurn, Kerri Peterson, Annette Polcino, and Stephanie Trentacoste. Without them my colleagues and I would not have been able to conduct this intensive two-year, longitudinal project.

It is my pleasure to thank all of the editors at New Harbinger Publications. The idea of this book was born of some lengthy conversations with Catharine Sutker, acquisitions editor. She not only encouraged me to write this book, she also provided invaluable encouragement throughout the process. My editor, Karen O'Donnell Stein, has been an unfailing source of enthusiasm as well. Her sensitivity and her ability to grasp and rework many of the concepts that I was trying to share with my readers made our working relationship a pleasure. If I write any books in the future, I will definitely call upon Karen O'Donnell Stein for her expertise. I must say that I think that I have a very striking book cover, and I thank Amy Shoup, art director, for her sophisticated, inviting cover design. And Heather Garnos, editorial manager, has been a reassuring presence as she directed the manuscript through the publication process with quiet competence.

Some of the research shared in this book was originally supported by several funding sources at the College of the Holy Cross, specifically the Howard Hughes Summer Research Fellowship Awards, Marshall Memorial Fund, and Holy Cross Student Research

Funds. I am grateful to the College of the Holy Cross for its ongoing support of my research.

There is no way to adequately thank the women who gave so generously of themselves and their time in talking with my research assistants and me about their struggles with sleep at various points in their lives. Without them, my book would not be the same. I hope that I have honored not just the content of their words, but the spirit in which they spoke with us. I thank them very much.

I also thank my colleague and close personal friend, Michaele McGinnes, for her support, ongoing inspiration, and her expertise regarding working with women who struggle with fibromyalgia, and other health problems that interfere with getting a good night's sleep.

Kathryn Lee, R.N., Ph.D., professor of Family Health Care Nursing, University of California, San Francisco School of Nursing, deserves special recognition. First of all, I thank Kathy for writing such an exciting and insightful foreword for my book. But, more importantly, I thank her for the historic contributions that she has made to research on women's sleep over the years. There would be no field of women's sleep if it were not for Dr. Lee's initial and ongoing research on women's sleep over the life span.

I want to thank Noah, my son, whose special friendship, understanding, and energy has made it possible for me to work on this long-term book project. I also thank you, Noah, for your wonderful sleep habits—something that mothers (fathers too) never take for granted.

I would also like to thank my father, Nicholas Wolfson, for his support of my career over many years, and for his advice as an author himself. I am lucky to have such an admirer in a father.

Last, but surely not least, there is my husband, Andy Futterman. As always, he has intimately shared my triumphs and pains in writing this book. He rejoiced with me when it was going well, encouraged me when I was sleep deprived and frustrated, and planned and cooked gourmet meals for all of us when I was too distracted to remember that we all needed to eat as well as sleep. He is not only my partner in life, my companion, and my colleague in the psychology department at Holy Cross; he is also, in the deepest sense, my very best friend.

Introduction to Sleep and Women's Health

Welcome to *The Women's Book of Sleep: A Complete Resource Guide*. Historically, women's health care was focused on maternal and child health, and medical research excluded women from important clinical trials which left significant gaps in understanding women's health concerns in areas such as heart disease, pharmacology, mental health, and sleep. But the publication of the book *Our Bodies, Ourselves*, in 1973, inspired many women to act as advocates for their own health needs. Then in 1991, the National Institutes of Health (NIH) launched a campaign to expand the involvement of women and minorities in clinical trials and initiated clinical research on women's midlife health concerns—osteoporosis, menopause, and hormone replacement therapy. Women's health is now a national priority.

Sleep is as important as nutrition and exercise throughout a woman's life, but it is often overlooked by health-care providers and women themselves. Although a number of excellent books have been written for women regarding mental and physical well-being, sleep has not been included in such self-help books, nor has it been given much attention in resource guides for health-care providers. I have focused much of my research and clinical career on sleep and daytime functioning, but often my friends and I do not have time to discuss how to improve or to increase the value of sleep in our lives. Despite our tendency to ignore it, sleep can make a big difference in our ability to function and feel good. One woman friend summed up the impact of sleep on her life: "I feel as if I can monitor how I am feeling about different aspects of my life—for example, work or family—by my sleep. Sleep is like a barometer for how I feel. I have no trouble falling asleep, but [when I'm under stress] I wake up in the middle of the night or very early in the morning."

As a sleep researcher and clinical psychologist, I am frequently asked questions about sleep needs, dreams, and sleep problems. Some commonly asked questions:

Why do I have such trouble getting to sleep?

Why haven't I had a good night's sleep since my children were born?

How can I make it so that my job doesn't interfere with my sleep?

Do other women complain that their sleep is disrupted when they menstruate?

How can I find the time to nap, like my husband does?

Does menopause disrupt sleep?

Why am I so exhausted all the time?

Do you have any recommendations for my chronic insomnia?

Can women get sleep apnea?

How can I make time for sleep?

It has become clear to me that more and more women are seeking information about improving their sleep. In recent years, I have been asked to speak with women's groups as well as women's health-care providers regarding the issue of women's sleep. At a recent women's conference at my local community center, I gave a talk entitled "A Guide for Women's Sleep" to a standing-room-only crowd. I love speaking with these audiences, but this book will answer the questions of many more women and health-care providers than I can speak to in a given year.

The Women's Bureau of the U.S. Department of Labor reported in its 1994 survey, entitled *Working Women Count*, of over a quarter of a million women from diverse economic and cultural backgrounds that the majority of working women like their jobs but perceive that their work is undervalued, and that stress and fatigue is their number one problem. Although there are still unanswered questions regarding women's sleep-wake patterns and sleep needs and disorders, in the last decade more research on women's sleep and gender differences in sleep-wake patterns and disorders has been conducted. These studies provide an expanding picture of some of the sleep-related issues that are particularly relevant to women's well-being over the course of their lives.

The National Sleep Foundation's Women and Sleep Poll (1998) found that on average women ages thirty to sixty sleep only six hours and forty minutes during the workweek. In other words, many women seem to cut back on their sleep and ignore signs of fatigue, daytime sleepiness, and other effects of insufficient sleep. The way women (and men for that manner) sleep critically affects how they think, act, and feel during daytime hours. Likewise, daytime activities, changes in the environment, and individual factors can have a profound effect on sleeping patterns. Throughout their lives women are confronted with important physical, cognitive, emotional, and social change such as giving birth, attending college, going through menopause, and working in the business world. One of the primary and most-often-ignored aspects of women's lives to be affected by these changes is sleep. Obtaining an adequate amount of sleep and keeping a regular sleep-wake schedule is crucial for women and men. Yet, experiences unique to women, like the menstrual cycle, pregnancy, and menopause, can affect your sleep due to fluctuating hormones (estrogen and progesterone) and environmental factors.

This book is meant to be helpful to you in a variety of ways. First, it should provide ready answers to your questions about sleep regardless of your age, work schedule, or family situation. Second, this book can be read either cover to cover or one section at a time for specific information on subjects such as insomnia or sleep during pregnancy. (If you do skip around, read through the first two chapters before looking into the chapter that meets your individual needs.) Third, this book may become a resource that you return to at different points in your life.

Throughout the book, I use terms from the sleep and women's health fields. Because many of these terms may be unfamiliar to you, I have included a glossary at the end of the book. Finally, at the end of most chapters, you'll find Sleep-Smart Strategies, techniques you can use to improve your sleep patterns.

Chapter 1 presents an overview of normal adult sleep, including discussions of sleep patterns and sleep architecture. Also, developmental changes in sleep from adolescence through older adulthood are addressed. Chapters 2 through 5 discuss sleep and rhythms as they relate to women's bodies, life cycles, and daily lives. I review how sleep-wake patterns change during the menstrual cycle, pregnancy, postpartum period, and menopause, and I provide tips that may help you deal with sleep disruptions during these times. Chapter 6 is devoted to sleep-wake patterns as they relate to working mothers, an important topic indeed given that approximately 50 percent of women with children under the age of three work outside the home, resulting in sleep issues both for children and for their working mothers. Chapters 7 and 8 include information and treatment recommendations regarding two common sleep disorders, insomnia and sleep apnea. Often perceived as an exclusively middle-aged male disease, sleep apnea afflicts 25 percent of women over the age of sixty-five and the incidence increases significantly after age fifty. Furthermore, insomnia symptoms, such as difficulty falling asleep or staying asleep, are reported by over 50 percent of women, nearly twice the rate of occurrence in men. As some readers know, insomnia symptoms have significant impact on physical and psychological well-being, as well as daytime functioning. Chapters 9 and 10 discuss the relationships between sleep and both physical health and mental health. Pain associated with health problems such as fibromyalgia, migraines, endometriosis, which are more common in or affect only women, often interferes with sleep. I offer intervention strategies that may enhance sleep if you suffer from fibromyalgia, migraines, or related health problems. In chapter 10, I summarize our current knowledge on the complex relationship between sleep disorders and mental health problems (e.g., depression and anxiety disorders), since most mood and anxiety disorders are more common in women than in men. This chapter will focus largely on diagnostic concerns and treatment recommendations regarding depression and anxiety as they relate to sleep-wake patterns. Finally, in the conclusion, I summarize what is currently known about sleep and women, provide information on future directions for the field, and discuss our roles as women clients (of sleep clinics), clinicians, researchers, and advocates for our health-care needs. I have also included an appendix of resources regarding the treatment of and research on sleep disorders.

Good, restful, restorative sleep can improve our health, outlook, competence, and sense of well-being. It is my hope that the information offered in The Women's Book of Sleep will help you to thoroughly understand and successfully manage your sleep as you go through developmental stages and challenging times in your life.

Normal Sleep over the Life Span

Many people believe that not much happens during the night—at around 10:30 P.M. your head hits the pillow and you do not recall anything until you wake to the sound of your buzzing alarm or your eight-year-old's yell from the kitchen for a glass of chocolate milk and two waffles with syrup. In fact, we all used to believe that once you fell asleep that was pretty much it until you woke up again. However, in recent decades we have learned that sleep is a very exciting and complex process.

From birth through older adulthood, the nature of sleep—its quality and quantity—develops and changes. If you observed someone sleeping for two hours, you would first see the sleeper in a period of very quiet, deep sleep, with regular, deep breathing, followed by a period of dreaming sleep, with frequent muscle twitches and eye movement back and forth under the eyelids. Sleepers are far more active than we generally realize. Recognition of the sleep stages and familiarity with age-related changes, including factors that disrupt or interfere with these stages, are important to understanding the relationship between women's sleep and daytime functioning. In the sections below, I try to explain the technical and scientific aspects of measuring, studying, and understanding sleep. You may find that you understand your own sleep patterns better after reading and sleeping on this chapter.

Circadian Rhythms

One cannot write a book on sleep without discussing *circadian rhythms*, biological rhythms that span a twenty-four-hour period. A biological rhythm is defined as a changing physiological process that reoccurs at regular intervals. Internal clocks that control biological rhythms having periods of about the length of a day are called circadian, from the Latin *circa* (about) and *dies* (day). Both men and women have biological rhythms that cycle approximately every twenty-four hours. See Czeisler and Khalsa (2000) for a complete presentation of the human circadian timing system. In fact, more than one-hundred physiological and psychological processes occur on a twenty-four-hour cycle.

As described by Dr. J. Allen Hobson, *states,* such as sleep, are considered phases of biological rhythms (1989). A state is defined as any relatively unchanging set of physiological conditions. In particular, sleep is a state that has certain conditions (e.g., the sleeper shows relatively little movement, is usually lying down or relaxed, and has minimal sensitivity to sounds, smells, and sights) and occurs for a finite period of time periodically over the twenty-four hour cycle. The sleep state can be broken down into substates; for example, REM sleep is a state within the state of sleep since it has definite conditions (e.g., active brain, muscle tone inhibition, and obviously rapid eye movements) that are distinct from those of other states and recurs periodically for a finite length of time each night (Hobson 1989).

Human beings normally depend on cues such as alarm clocks, school bells, sunsets, meal times, and ambient temperature changes to tell us when to awake and when to sleep. However, research on circadian rhythms demonstrates that we are not just reacting to environmental cues, we are actually following internally generated rhythms. Studies have shown that twenty-four-hour rhythms of rest and activity, sleeping and waking, and body temperature persist even when time cues, referred to as *zeitgebers* (time givers), are removed.

Moreover, researchers have actually located the probable site of the circadian clock in the brain, specifically in the *hypothalamus*. The hypothalamus is a structure in the central part of the brain with many interconnections to other brain regions. The biological clock is located in the *suprachiasmatic nucleus* (SCN) within the hypothalamus, just above the optic chiasm, the point at which the nerves from the two eyes cross on their way to opposite sides of the brain (Moore and Eichler 1972). The SCN helps to coordinate the activity of the rest of the brain (and body) so as to bring it into harmony with daily cycles of environmental heat and light. So, what does all of this mean and why is it important in our discussion of women's sleep?

Evidently, there are two mechanisms that govern how alert or sleepy we feel at any given time in our twenty-four-hour cycle. First, we have a sort of sleep-wake balance, called a homeostatic system, whereby we feel either more alert or more sleepy depending on how long we have been awake relative to when and for how long we last slept. Second, we feel more sleepy or more alert depending on where we are in our twenty-four-hour circadian cycle. We feel most sleepy in the early dawn hours, in the late afternoon, and close to our bedtime. In contrast, generally we feel most alert in the morning and/or early afternoon, and again in the early evening hours.

Our sleep-wake homeostatic system, together with the circadian timing of sleep and activity, govern how we feel throughout the day. For example, both you and I may feel sleepy at about four o'clock in the afternoon and quite alert just before dinner regardless of how much we each slept the night before. However, if you have a more regular sleep-wake schedule and are obtaining an adequate amount of sleep while I have an irregular schedule and do not get enough sleep, you will usually feel more alert and energetic than I will.

* * * * *

I hope that you now have a good sense of what a normal sleep cycle is and how it changes over the course of your life. When you were a baby, your main jobs were to sleep, eat, and cry. Reaching adolescence, you still needed quite a lot of sleep, but your sleep schedule probably changed. Now, as an adult, you most likely sleep less than you did as a child. However, you probably have decided to read this book because you are not totally satisfied with the amount of sleep you are getting. Read on for some strategies that can help you get the sleep you need.

Your Night Flight: Sleep Architecture

During sleep, you repeatedly move through four stages of sleep, which are punctuated by brief awakenings. Although cycling between the various sleep stages is rather fluid, sleep researchers have established criteria to mark the beginnings and endings of the four stages. The stages of sleep are traditionally observed by recording changes in the sleeper's brain waves, eye movements, and muscle tension while they sleep in a research laboratory. (See *Principles and Practice of Sleep Medicine*, by Meir Kryger, Thomas Roth, and William Dement (2000), for a thorough review of basic adult sleep phenomena and mechanisms.) The changes are clearly not haphazard. Using recordings of our brain waves while we are awake and asleep (i.e., polysomnographic measures), sleep researchers have divided sleep into two major components: *Rapid Eye Movement* (REM) sleep and *non-Rapid Eye Movement* (NREM) sleep. NREM sleep is further divided into four stages of sleep. Stage 1, transitional sleep, is light sleep or drowsiness characterized by the following: slow, regular brain activity; slow, rolling, pendulous eye movements; slow, regular breathing; relaxed muscles; and minimal body movements. Some clinicians and researchers argue that this is not really sleep at all because you are still aware of what is going on around you; it's like a no-woman's-land, somewhere between sleep and wakefulness.

As you move more deeply into sleep, the pattern of your brain waves changes. They become slower, but occasionally bursts of faster rhythms occur. These are called *sleep spindles* because their pattern on the EEG takes the shape of a spindle on a spinning wheel. This indicates that you are now in Stage 2, the most frequently occurring stage of sleep, characterized by an absence of eye movements and moderate muscle activity. Both sleep spindles and *k-complexes* appear during Stage 2; the sleep spindles are bursts of 12 to 14 distinct and rhythmic EEG peaks and valleys per second and k-complexes are sudden, high-amplitude bipolar spikes. Traditionally, sleep researchers use the first sleep spindle or k-complex as the marker for the onset of sleep. If you were to awaken at this point, you would probably report having been asleep. It is unlikely that you would recall any dreams, but you might report having had some fragmented thoughts.

Next, much larger waves appear, indicating Stages 3 and 4, which are characterized by deep sleep with very regular respiration and minimal response to the environment. Stages 3 and 4 sleep is often referred to as delta sleep or *slow-wave sleep* (SWS) because of the shapes made on an EEG when these stages are being recorded.

When you initially fall asleep, you go through all four of these NREM sleep stages in sequence. Then, after about 90 to 110 minutes, there is a dramatic change. The brain waves speed up suddenly and look similar to those of a waking state, just not quite as fast. The eyes are closed, but every now and then they move suddenly from side to side. To the observer (perhaps a parent watching his or her baby or a sleep lab technician monitoring a patient), it looks like the person is watching a video on an invisible screen in front of them. These movements, discovered and named by Dr. Nathaniel Kleitman, and Dr. Eugene Aserinsky, in 1953, are called Rapid Eye Movements (REM).

REM is often referred to as dreaming sleep because 80 to 90 percent of dreaming occurs during REM sleep. REM is characterized as a period of intense brain activity with rapid eye movements, irregular respiration and heart rate, and dreaming. During REM sleep, most of your muscles are nearly paralyzed, which prevents you from acting out your dreams. However, a rare sleep disorder, REM Sleep Behavior Disorder (RBD), causes complex and violent behaviors to emerge during REM sleep, when ordinarily muscles are nearly paralyzed. People with RBD will attempt to act out their nightmares while asleep, unaware of their surroundings. RBD typically affects older men. Fortunately, this disorder can be controlled using medication.

The process described above, the four sleep stages followed by a period of REM sleep, constitutes a sleep cycle, and it is repeated every 90 to 110 minutes throughout a typical night of seven to ten hours of sleep. This first period of REM sleep follows the four stages of NREM sleep. On average, you will have between four and six complete sleep cycles each night. The first REM period usually lasts about 10 minutes, but as the night progresses, the NREM periods become shorter and the REM periods become longer. In total REM occupies approximately 90 to 120 minutes of sleep each night. SWS usually occurs only in the first one or two cycles of the night and tends to decrease during adulthood.

Most adults spend approximately 80 percent of the night in NREM sleep and 20 percent in REM sleep. Both NREM and REM sleep are equally important and beneficial, and your body will do what it can to make sure you get sleep in the right order and in the right proportion. Although you manage the amount and timing of your sleep, you cannot consciously control the order of your sleep stages. It is your nervous system that controls and balances your sleep stages. For example, if you are deprived of REM sleep for a few nights (e.g., from taking a medication that suppresses REM or sleeping only three to four hours each night for several days while taking care of a sick child), your brain will generate more REM sleep at the next opportunity (such as when you're at the movies on a Saturday night).

Sleep Need

So, how much sleep do most adult women need? Like many women, you probably worry about whether or not you are getting enough sleep. According to sleep researchers, the amount of sleep needed by the average adult is 7.5 to 8 hours each night. Studies have documented that adults' self-reported total sleep time ranges from 4.5 to 10.5 hours (Webb 1992). It has also been reported that the average amount of sleep on workdays was about 7.5 hours for both male and female shift workers. On days off the average for males was 9 hours, 7 minutes; for females it was less, 8 hours, 53 minutes (Webb 1985). Similarly, sleep researchers Mary Carskadon and William Dement

(1994) reported that most adults sleep approximately 7.5 hours on weekdays and 8.5 hours on weekends.

However, women do not seem to be obtaining an adequate amount of sleep. In a 1995 survey of nearly two hundred women ages twenty-two to fifty-eight (see chapter 6), their average total weeknight sleep time was found to be only about 7 hours. More recently, sleep expert Thomas Wehr (1991) examined adults' sleep needs in a laboratory setting. Wehr and colleagues kept adults on a 10-14-hour light-dark schedule (a 10-hour night and a 14-hour day) for several weeks. After many nights of greater than 9 or 10 hours of sleep, the sleep quotients of these adults' leveled off at approximately 8 hours, 23 minutes. Wehr's studies demonstrate that the old hypothesis that adults need only 7 to 8 hours of sleep each night may be inaccurate.

Nevertheless, it is crucial to remember that this 8 hours is an average amount, and the amount of sleep needed varies from woman to woman, and from one developmental stage to another. Misconceptions regarding sleep need and recommended sleep habits may create problems and worries. For example, many people believe that once they go to sleep they don't wake up until morning; however, it's normal for adults and children to briefly awaken approximately every 90 minutes, four to five times each night, as you cycle through the sleep stages that I described earlier. To help you understand some of these misconceptions and avoid unnecessary worries over your sleep, I discuss sleep need and recommended sleep-wake habits throughout the book, particularly in the chapter on insomnia.

Developmental Changes in Sleep-Wake Patterns

Sleep quality and quantity changes throughout our lives. You may look at your infant, as she zones out periodically throughout the day and envy her ability to drift off at any time. But sleeping is a newborn's main job. Specifically, a critical task of the newborn infant is to organize behavior into specific states—awake, NREM, and REM sleep—and to organize these states into a twenty-four-hour rhythmic pattern. Infants' sleep states are not as clearly demarcated as adults' sleep states are. Three sleep states can be identified in the newborn: *active sleep* (REM), *quiet sleep* (NREM), and *indeterminate sleep*. Indeterminate sleep is defined as a state in which characteristics of neither REM nor NREM can be identified. Indeterminate sleep, or transitional sleep, diminishes over the course of the first year. Obviously, infants' and toddlers' sleep cycles differ from those of adults. An infant's sleep cycle is shorter than an adult's (fifty minutes versus ninety minutes). In addition, during the first three to six months, REM sleep decreases markedly. At age three months, the infant spends 50 percent of her sleep period in REM and 50 percent in NREM; by the time she reaches adulthood she will spend only 20 percent of the night in REM. This decreasing amount of REM sleep is considered a critical indicator of central nervous system development.

One of the most obvious changes during a child's first five years is the amount of time she spends sleeping each day. On average, total sleep time decreases over these early years from about seventeen to eleven hours. At six or seven weeks of age, babies begin to spend more time sleeping at night and less during the day; however, it is not until they reach approximately three months of age that daytime sleep is differentiated from nighttime sleep. Then, sometime between six and nine months, most babies settle into a pattern of well-consolidated nighttime sleep. From approximately six to seven years of age to the beginning of adolescence, total sleep decreases slightly, from about ten hours to about nine hours.

In adolescents, sleep structure or architecture is similar to that of adults. The key changes in sleep-wake patterns and requirements associated with puberty for both young men and women are striking: Although adolescents require at least as much sleep as they did as preadolescents (in general 8.5 to 9.25 hours per night), their sleep patterns undergo a phase delay, meaning a tendency to go to sleep and wake up later. And even when a teenager gets an optimal amount of sleep, she is still likely to report experiencing greater daytime sleepiness than she did when she was younger. (My colleagues and I have written extensively on teens and sleep see "Sleep Schedules and Daytime Functioning in Adolescents" [Wolfson and Carskadon 1998].)

The changes in sleep beyond adolescence, into the twenties and thirties, are less remarkable. Between the ages of six and eighteen, the total amount of sleep gradually declines from about eleven hours to about eight to nine hours.

Aging and Sleep

Sleep-wake patterns also change as we get older. You may have assumed that you will need less and less sleep as you celebrate significant birthdays—forty, fifty, sixty, seventy, and so on. Actually, as we get older we probably need just as much sleep. Yet, the pattern of sleeping changes with age. In comparison to twenty-year-old, a sixty-year-old has more awakenings each night (on average six per night as opposed to one per night). Also, although those in the sixty-plus set are likely to sleep for shorter periods, they are also more likely to nap or snooze, while watching the evening news, for example. Light sleep (Stage 1) is 2.5 times as great in the sixty-year-old. Although REM sleep and Stage 2 sleep barely change between ages twenty and sixty, deep sleep (Stage 4) diminishes by 15 to 30 percent. However, there are tremendous individual differences in the response of sleep to age. Some of you will experience far fewer changes in your sleep patterns over the years in comparison to some of your friends. See chapters 2 through 5 for discussion regarding some of the specific changes that women may experience at various life stages.

Sleep-Smart Strategies

Below are general sleep hygiene recommendations—use these to improve the overall quality and quantity of your sleep.

* Keep regular hours. The best way to ensure perfect nights is to stick to a regular schedule. If you sleep late one morning and rise before dawn the next, you can come down with an at-home version of jet lag. To keep your biological clock on a regular rhythm, get up at the same time every day, regardless of how much or how little you've slept. Try to stick to your usual sleep schedule on weekends and holidays as well as on workdays. If you stay up late on Friday and Saturday nights and sleep in the following mornings, you may give yourself a case of "Sunday-night insomnia," meaning that despite going to bed early on Sunday night (to be well rested Monday morning), you just can not sleep—the harder you try, the more wakeful you feel. So when travel, work, or recreation throws off your routine, try to maintain a modicum of regularity. Eat your meals at the same times you normally do. Try to get some sleep during your usual bedtime hours. And return to your normal schedule as soon as you can.

* Exercise regularly. Exercise burns off the tensions that accumulate during the day, allowing both body and mind to unwind. Although the fit seem to sleep better and deeper than the flabby, you do not have to push to utter exhaustion. A twenty- to thirty-minute walk, jog, swim, or bicycle ride at least three days a week—the minimum needed to achieve cardiovascular benefits—should be your goal. Do not exercise right before bedtime, and do not wait until very late in the day to exercise. In the evening you should be concentrating on winding down rather than on working up a sweat. Early-morning exercise is great for boosting your energy, but it doesn't have any impact on the tensions that build up during the day. The ideal exercise time is late afternoon or early evening, when your workout can help you shift gears from daytime pressures to evening pleasures.

* Cut down on stimulants. North Americans drink 400 million cups of coffee a day and get extra doses of caffeine in tea, soft drinks, and chocolate. Some people seem sensitive to even small amounts; others build up a tolerance. If you're a coffee or cola lover, have your last caffeinated beverage of the day no later than six to eight hours before your bedtime. Its stimulating effects will peak two to four hours after you drink it, although they'll linger for several hours more. Late-evening caffeine can make it harder for you to fall asleep, diminish deep sleep, and increase nighttime awakenings. And caffeine is not the only dietary sleep-robber. *Tyrosine*, a substance found in chocolate, Chianti, and cheddar cheese can trigger heart palpitations in the night. Diet pills contain stimulants that can keep you awake. Other drugs or drug interactions can also disrupt your nights. If you're taking any prescription or over-the-counter drugs, ask your health-care provider whether they could affect your sleep.

* Sleep on good bedding. Just as you need good running shoes to run well, you need good bedding to sleep well. Good bedding helps you fall asleep and stay asleep, and it prevents damage to your back and neck while you sleep. Start with a good mattress. Select some good, new pillows, which are adjustable for healthy support and comfortable sleep. Finally, snuggle up under a comforter—down is lighter and will keep you more comfortable than will conventional bedding.

* Do not smoke. Nicotine is an even stronger stimulant than caffeine. According to several studies, heavy smokers take longer to fall asleep, awaken more often, and spend less time in REM and deep NREM sleep. Because nicotine withdrawal can start two to three hours after the last puff, some smokers awake in the night craving a cigarette. When smokers break their nicotine addiction, their sleep improves dramatically after a few weeks: in one study, two-pack-a-day smokers who quit cut the time they lay awake in bed by almost half.

* Drink only in moderation. Alcohol is the oldest, most popular sleep aid. Although having a nightcap is a habit for many, consuming liquor late in the evening may cause problems throughout the night. Even moderate drinking can suppress REM and deep NREM sleep and accelerate shifts between sleep stages. Taking too much alcohol with dinner can make it harder to fall asleep and having too much at bedtime can make it harder to stay asleep. As the immediate effects of the alcohol wear off, REM sleep—which alcohol suppresses—intrudes upon other sleep

stages, depriving your body of deep rest. You end up sleeping in fragments and waking often in the early-morning hours.

* Do your planning for the next day early in the evening. If you find that you often lie in bed thinking about what you should have done during the day or what you have to do the next day, try to deal with such distractions before getting into bed. Make lists so you do not feel you have to keep reminding yourself of the things you need to do. Write out anxieties or worries and possible solutions. If daytime distractions still follow you into bed, tell yourself that you'll deal with them during the next day.

* Do not go to bed stuffed or starved. Eating a big meal late at night forces your digestive system to work overtime. While you may feel drowsy initially, you'll probably toss and turn through the night. Avoid foods that can cause gas, such as peanuts, beans, and certain fruits or raw vegetables. And stay away from snacks that are high in fat—they take longer to digest. If you're dieting, don't go to bed hungry. A rumbling stomach, like any other physical discomfort, interferes with your ability to settle down and slumber through the night. If you're hungry, have a low-calorie snack, such as a banana or an apple, before turning in.

* Develop a bedtime ritual. Before you can slide into sleep, you've got to leave behind the distractions of the waking world. Even very young children find it easier to make the transition into sleep if they repeat the same activities, such as saying prayers or reading a story, every night. Your sleep ritual can be as simple or elaborate as you choose.

  You might start by doing some gentle stretches to release knots of tension in your muscles or with a warm bath, followed by listening to some quiet music or curling up with a not-too-thrilling book. Whatever you choose, try to do the same things every evening until they become cues for your body to settle down for the night.

* 2 *

Understanding Your Menstrual Cycle and Sleep Patterns

Even with my eyes shut and my head in the pillow, I know that it is the middle of the night. Why am I acutely aware of everything? Am I getting cramps? What did I eat last night? Is my son up? Should I just get out of bed and get some work done? Did I call my father? Why am I so restless and uncomfortable? I finally check the clock; it is 4:26 A.M. and I am positive that I will be a wreck in the morning. Does this scenario sound familiar?

Sex Differences in Sleep

Women are twice as likely to complain of insufficient and poor sleep than men, according to a number of questionnaire and interview studies of young to middle-aged men and women (Lugaresi, Cirginotta, Zucconi, Mondini, Lenzi, and Coccagna 1983). In addition, women report a greater need for sleep, greater daytime sleepiness, longer total sleep times, more trouble maintaining sleep, and greater consumption of sleeping tablets than men do, whereas men report that it takes them longer to fall asleep (including my own husband, who complains an awful lot about his poor sleep and his difficulties falling asleep). (Jacquinet-Salord, Lang, Fouriaud, Nicoulet, and Bingham 1993) It is noteworthy, however, that women often attribute their poor sleep to psychological factors, while men blame their sleeping difficulties on work-related issues (Urponen, Vuori, Hasan, and Partinen 1988).

Other studies have examined sex differences in the architecture of sleep. It appears, according to a small number of studies, that a few sex differences in sleep architecture do exist. A relatively recent study demonstrated that slow-wave sleep (SWS) decreases at a later age in women than in men (Ehlers and Kupfer 1997). Studies are beginning to assess the influence of estrogen, progesterone, and other hormones on women's sleep.

This chapter is focused on the sleep-wake pattern changes that occur in many women over the course of their menstrual cycles. For example, recent research concludes that during menstruation women tend to get less restful sleep, and that after ovulation (i.e., when progesterone levels begin to decrease) some women find it more difficult to fall asleep.

The Menstrual Cycle

As you read through this section, you may find it helpful to refer to the diagram on the next page. Let's review what really happens during your menstrual cycle. (See *Our Bodies, Ourselves*, by the Boston Women's Health Collective, 1998, for a thorough review of the menstrual cycle.) Ninety percent of women under forty-five years of age menstruate regularly; by age fifty-five, just 10 percent menstruate regularly (Lee and Taylor 1996). Most women's menstrual cycles are twenty-eight days long, but some of your cycles may be as short as twenty-one days or as long as thirty-five days. Some women have alternating short and long cycles. The length of a woman's menstrual cycle (the number of days from the first day of one period to the first day of the next) is determined by the number of days that it takes her ovary to release an egg. Ovulation occurs about fourteen to sixteen days before a menstrual period begins, but its timing changes from woman to woman and across cycles. The second half of the cycle, ovulation to menstruation, is fairly consistent in length.

Your monthly menstrual period is actually the result of a complex physiological process. First, the brain's hypothalamus gland, responsible for regulating the body's thirst, hunger, sleep, libido, and endocrine functions, releases *Follicle Stimulating Hormone Releasing Factor* (FSH-RF). FSH-RF informs the pituitary gland to begin the process. The pituitary then secretes *Follicle Stimulating Hormone* (FSH) and *Leutenizing Hormone* (LH) into the bloodstream, causing the eggs stored in the follicles, located in the ovaries, to begin to mature.

The maturing follicles then release another hormone, estrogen. As the follicles mature over about five to seven days, they secrete increasingly more estrogen into the bloodstream. The estrogen causes the lining of the uterus to thicken and cervical mucus to

MENSTRUAL CYCLE CLOCK

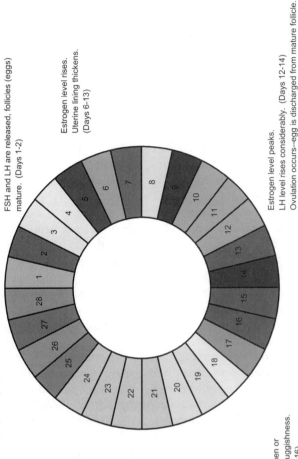

Hypothalamus releases FSH-RF and bleeding begins. (Day 1)

FSH and LH are released, follicles (eggs) mature. (Days 1-2)

Estrogen level rises. Uterine lining thickens. (Days 6-13)

Estrogen level peaks. LH level rises considerably. (Days 12-14) Ovulation occurs--egg is discharged from mature follicle.

Possible cramping in lower abdomen or back, headaches, gastric pains, sluggishness. Conception most likely. (Days 14-16)

Basal body temperature rises. (Days 14-18)

Estrogen and progesterone are released if conception has not occurred. (Days 14-22)

Progesterone peaks. (Days 21-22)

Symptoms of PMS or Late Luteal Phase Dysphoric Disorder. (Days 22-28)

Bloating, backache, headaches, breast tenderness, irritability, nausea. (Days 24-28)

Sleep most disturbed--insomnia, daytime tiredness, difficulty waking, nighttime awakenings. (Days 24-28)

Arthritis, digestive tract disorders, fibromyalgia, migraines, skin conditions flare. (Day 25-Day 2)

Estrogen and progesterone levels drop. Arteries and veins in uterus close off. Endometrium breaks down. (Day 27-Day 1) change. Once a woman's estrogen level reaches a certain point, *Leutenizing Hormone Releasing Factor* (LH-RF) causes the pituitary to release a considerable amount of LH. At this point, about mid-cycle, ovulation occurs: the egg is discharged out of the most mature follicle (*corpus luteum*) and from the surface of the ovary, to be received by the fallopian tube. As ovulation occurs, the blood supply to the ovary increases and the ligaments supporting the uterus contract to pull the ovary closer to the fallopian tube. At this time, many of you may have cramping in the lower abdomen or back, and a few women experience headaches, gastric pains, or sluggishness; others may feel quite good at the time of ovulation. Basal body temperature rises right after ovulation and remains elevated until a few days before menstruation.

If the egg becomes fertilized, the ovum travels to the uterine cavity and embeds itself in the *endometrium* (uterine lining) and starts its growth. If it does not become fertilized (i.e., conception does not occur), the follicle from which the egg was released, or corpus luteum, will produce estrogen and progesterone in gradually decreasing amounts for about twelve days. As the estrogen and progesterone levels drop, the tiny arteries and veins in the uterus close off. As a result, the endometrium breaks down and menstruation occurs for an average of four to six days.

As you know, women may experience a variety of symptoms before, during, and after their period. Common complaints include cramping, backache, bloating, nausea, gastrointestinal problems (diarrhea, constipation, or indigestion), headaches (specifically migraines), breast tenderness, irritability, and other mood changes. Cramping, spasmodic and congestive, is one of the most common menstrual symptoms. Spasmodic cramping is related to the *prostaglandins*, chemicals that affect muscle tension, and congestive cramping occurs when the body retains fluids and salt.

Menstrual Effects on Sleep

Observably, adolescent and adult women experience cyclical changes in reproductive hormone levels. Interestingly, research suggests that premenopausal women's endocrine systems may actually buffer them against stress, activate their immune systems, and improve their cardiovascular health. Because of changing women's hormone levels, both monthly and throughout the life span, women have often been excluded from research on sleep, circadian rhythms, and other sleep-related factors. Fortunately, this has changed over the last decade; in the section below, I highlight the recent crucial findings regarding our menstrual cycles and sleep.

According to the National Sleep Foundation's Women and Sleep Poll (1998), in which over one thousand women ages thirty to sixty were interviewed, the menstrual cycle, pregnancy, and menopause can affect sleep. Specifically, 25 to 50 percent of the women surveyed reported that menstruation symptoms (bloating, tender breasts, headaches, and cramps/pain) disturb their sleep for approximately two to three days of their cycle. Many of the women also reported other sleep difficulties during menstruation, including taking longer to fall asleep, waking at night and being unable to fall back to sleep, feeling less refreshed in the morning, having difficulty getting out of bed in the morning, and waking earlier. Nearly 70 percent of the women surveyed felt sleepiest the week prior to or during the first few days of their period. One woman explained:

> Since the age of forty, my sleep has been very disrupted during my menstrual cycle. During menstruation, I feel so exhausted that I need to retire much earlier than usual, and during midcycle each month, I need to go to bed at around eight o'clock when my children go to sleep.

Still, women's sleep experiences vary greatly during the menstrual cycle. Some women may not have any changes in their sleep, whereas others experience premenstrual hypersomnia, a rare sleep disorder that causes excessive daytime somnolence in association with menstruation.

We can now begin to draw conclusions regarding sleep changes over the course of the menstrual cycle, from information gathered in studies conducted during the 1980s and 1990s (Driver and Baker 1998). The sleep changes that you and other women may experience over the course of your menstrual cycle can be linked to increasing and decreasing hormone levels.

Women report that they experience longer sleep latencies (the time it takes to fall asleep), reduced sleep quality, and daytime sleepiness during the late luteal phase (after ovulation) in comparison to the mid-follicular phase of their menstrual cycles (Manber and Bootzin 1997). After ovulation, progesterone levels start off high and begin to decrease toward the end of this phase. Your difficulty falling asleep, your feeling that your sleep is less restful, and/or your excessive daytime sleepiness or lethargy after ovulation and at the beginning of menstruation may be related to these rapidly falling levels of progesterone. In fact, progesterone can be as sedating as sleeping pills, and some research suggests that the more quickly and sharply your hormone levels fall at the end of your cycle, the more you may toss and turn during the night. Dr. Helen Driver and her colleagues demonstrated that elevated body temperature in the post-ovulatory phase of the menstrual cycle may disrupt sleep stages and structure, specifically resulting in decreased REM sleep quantity (Driver, Dijk, Werth, Biedermann, and Borbely 1996). However, several noteworthy laboratory studies found that women without self-reported changes in their sleep did not show any significant variation in the length of time it took them to fall asleep, in the length of time until their first Rapid Eye Movement (REM) episode, or in the amount of slow-wave sleep (SWS) (Lee, Shaver, Giblin, and Woods 1990). Dr. Helen Driver and her colleagues also demonstrated that elevated body temperature in the postovulatory phase of the menstrual cycle may disrupt sleep stages and structure, specifically resulting in decreased REM sleep quantity (Driver, Dijk, Werth, Biedermann, and Borbely 1996).

Premenstrual Syndrome (PMS)

Premenstrual Syndrome (PMS) symptoms may occur during the later portion of this phase (starting in the week or two preceding a menstrual period). Eighty percent of women of reproductive age experience some emotional or behavioral changes when they are premenstrual, but PMS symptoms occur in only about 5 to 10 percent of women. The symptoms include bloating, headaches, moodiness, irritability, and abdominal cramps.

Women who experience PMS may be at particular risk for sleep difficulties. Recent studies have shown that women with definitive PMS show different polysomnographic brain recordings than do women without PMS. In a study that compared these two groups of women, the researcher found that women who suffer from PMS experienced significantly less deep, restorative sleep (Stages 3 and 4) not only before their periods, when progesterone plummets, but during the entire month. Specifically, a healthy sleeper spends about 15 to 20 percent of his or her sleep time in deep sleep. Research suggests that women who suffer from PMS experience less deep sleep (about 5 percent of their total sleep) all month long. The most common sleep-related problems reported by women who experience PMS are: insomnia (difficulty falling asleep, difficulty staying asleep, or waking up too early), hypersomnia (sleeping too much), unpleasant dreams, difficulty waking up in the morning, and morning and daytime tiredness.

Dysmenorrhea

Women who suffer from dysmenorrhea regularly experience painful menstrual cramps that disrupt their personal lives. Primary dysmenorrhea occurs in the absence of any identifiable pelvic pathology and is not explained by stress or other psychological factors. Although the exact cause is unclear, prostaglandins may mediate the pain. It is not surprising that women with dysmenorrhea report fatigue and disturbed sleep due to uterine cramps; they experience lower sleep efficiency (amount of time asleep relative to the amount of time in bed), spend greater time in Stage 1 sleep and wakefulness than do women who are free of menstrual cramps. Also, women with dysmenorrhea have decreased REM sleep and higher nocturnal body temperatures.

Endometriosis

Without a doubt, endometriosis may interfere with the ability to fall asleep and maintain sleep throughout the night. Endometriosis is a condition affecting approximately 5 million women (including myself) in the United States and Canada in which the tissue lining the inside of the uterus appears elsewhere in the pelvis, in or around areas such as the abdomen, ovaries, fallopian tubes, and ligaments that support the uterus (Domar and Dreher 1996).

Other sites for these endometrial growths may include the bladder, bowel, vagina, cervix, vulva, and in abdominal surgical scars. This misplaced tissue develops into growths or lesions that respond to the menstrual cycle in the same way that the tissue of the uterine lining does. Specifically, each month the tissue builds up, breaks down, and sheds. Tissue shed from endometrial growths has no way of leaving the body, and this results in internal bleeding, breakdown of the blood and tissue from the lesions, and inflammation, causing pain, infertility, scar-tissue formation, adhesions, and bowel problems. The most commons symptoms are pain before and during periods; painful sexual experiences; infertility; daytime sleepiness; discomfort of the urinary tract and bowels during periods; and other gastrointestinal upsets such as diarrhea, constipation, and nausea. The stress and pain associated with endometriosis contribute to sleep difficulties and, as a result, daytime sleepiness. Diagnosis is considered most certain when proven through laparoscopy, a minor surgical procedure done under anesthesia (Endometriosis Association 2000).

To date, the exact cause of endometriosis has not been found. Yet, researchers do know that estrogen promotes endometrial overgrowth in some women, and the fact that many women are having children at older ages and, therefore, are having more menstrual cycles before their first pregnancy may explain the increasing prevalence of endometriosis (Domar and Dreher 1996). Other researchers argue that stress may contribute to the progression and exacerbation of the symptoms (Lauersen and DeSwann 1988).

If you are experiencing endometriosis, you should consult a gynecologist or other health-care provider to discuss the medical treatments available. Unfortunately, there is no magical solution for treating endometriosis. On the other hand, a number of mind-body approaches are often beneficial for women with chronic or inter-mittent pain caused by endometriosis or other conditions (e.g., fibromyalgia and migraines; see chapter 9). For example, you may want to try keeping a pain diary (Caudill 1994), utilizing progressive relaxation (see appendix B), and other behavioral approaches to pain and sleep hygiene.

Sleep-Smart Strategies during Menstruation

Women have been sharing menstrual remedies for centuries. Now it may be time to focus on improving your sleep during various points in your menstrual cycle. Listed below are strategies that women like you have reported as beneficial or that research studies have demonstrated as effective. I am sure that you will find that some strategies work better than others for you; however, none of the strategies will work unless you try them in a consistent, regular fashion. If you experience PMS, you may find these suggestions par-ticularly helpful.

* Allow enough time for sleep. Obtaining an adequate amount of sleep throughout the month, particularly during menstruation, helps to cushion you during the times when you may have diffi-culty falling or remaining asleep. Your circadian rhythms may change during your cycle. Try to allow extra time for sleep at night if you tend to experience excessive daytime sleepiness or other changes in your sleep quality. For example, ask your spouse or partner to put the children to bed, so you can get to bed early, or ask them to get up with your toddler if she wakes up during the night. If at all possible, plan to take a brief nap on the days that you feel particularly sleepy or drained (although I realize this may seem like an impossible suggestion).

* Exercise in moderation regularly. Exercise may relieve some PMS symptoms and increase your amount of deep sleep (Stages 3, 4). But be sure to complete your workout at least three hours before your bedtime.

* Avoid caffeine. Having caffeine in the evening disturbs sleep—even in those people who thinks it does not affect them. I cannot tell you the number of times that my close friends, family members, and, of course, college students emphatically have said to me that they are not at all affected by caffeine, even those who have trouble sleeping! Caffeine is found in coffee, tea (both iced and hot), chocolate, sodas, and even some specialty bottled waters. Caffeine takes six to eight hours for your body to metabolize and therefore you should avoid these stimulant drinks after lunchtime. Caffeinated beverages may also increase premenstrual bloating and therefore worsen your already disrupted sleep. (See appendix B for more information on caffeine.)

* Avoid alcohol. Drinking alcohol may help you to fall asleep easily in the evening, but it also results in fragmented sleep, particularly over the second half of the sleep period. Women (and men) who drink alcohol to assist with sleep onset generally obtain less total nighttime sleep than they would if they abstained from alcohol. Also, alcohol, like caffeine, can increase premenstrual bloating and disrupt sleep.

* Avoid large meals and excessive fluid intake. Taken before bedtime, these may cause poor sleep, indigestion, heartburn, or frequent awakenings to urinate. Bedtime snacks should be small and consist of non-spicy foods.

* Evaluate your use of nonsteroidal anti-inflammatory drugs (NSAIDs), such as ibuprofen. Some of you will find that NSAIDs help relieve menstrual cramps just before and during your period. Obviously, if you are more comfortable, you will be likely to fall asleep and remain asleep during the night. Indeed, a number of studies have demonstrated that NSAIDs decrease PMS symptoms, particularly cramps, headaches, and dizziness (Mortola 1994; Wood and Jakubowicz 1980). Unfortunately, however, NSAIDs often bring on stomach upset and other gastrointestinal difficulties.

* 3 *

Sleep Patterns during Pregnancy

Nearly fifteen years ago, while I was conducting a study on infant sleep, I began meeting with expectant mothers and fathers to recruit them to participate in a study on infants' sleeping patterns. They were thrilled to participate, but many of the women laughed and commented that I should really be studying their sleep! Their words sparked my interest. So, more recently, I set out to conduct a study on women's sleep during pregnancy and early motherhood. I found that my expectant friends, colleagues, and study participants were thrilled that someone was finally listening to their sleep complaints, needs, and changes during this milestone period in their lives.

In my longitudinal study, *Sleep and Mood from the Last Trimester of Pregnancy through Twelve Months Postpartum* (Wolfson and Anser 2000), a number of women shared their experiences with me. Their stories will probably be familiar to you. Below are three women's comments:

> During the entire length of my third trimester, I just could not sleep well. I was constantly tired during the day and night, but when it was time to go to bed it took forever to get comfortable. Throughout the night, I was awakened by cramps, the need to use the bathroom, and sometimes my baby's kicking movements. Although I was exhausted, I would wake up before my alarm clock because of one of these disturbances. Some nights, I lay awake thinking about all of the things that I had to accomplish before my due date.
>
> I was exhausted. I was into my eighth hour of labor and I truly felt I had no more energy. The last two weeks leading up to this day were exhausting as well. Into the fifteenth hour, my

nurse-midwife and partner were coaching me to keep up my strength, but they did not seem to understand that it was three in the morning. At 5:30 A.M., after seventeen and one-half hours of labor, I held my son in my arms. I started to doze off with him in my arms just as my parents arrived to see their first grandson. After a couple of hours of showing off baby David, I was finally able to sleep.

At two in the morning, Beth was crying to be fed. I, choosing to breastfeed, had to be the one to go feed her. This was the third time this evening that Beth had awakened for some reason. In the two weeks since Beth was born, my longest stretch of sleep had been about four hours. After nursing Beth, I changed her and, an hour after getting up, I was back in bed. I groaned as I looked at the clock and realized that my husband's alarm would buzz momentarily. During the day, I tried to nap when Beth did, but there was so much to do. In about six weeks, I was supposed to return to work full-time. I was stressed about the thought of working and being a mother on this minimal amount of sleep.

Pregnancy, childbirth, and early motherhood can be some of the most joyous times in a woman's life, but this period also can be a time of great uncertainty and discomfort. As women, we are asked to balance the social, physical, and psychological changes that occur simultaneously from the very beginning of pregnancy throughout childbirth and into the postpartum period. In a recently published study, Dr. Jodi Mindell and colleagues (2000) found that 97 percent of pregnant women fail to sleep through the night by the end of their pregnancy and 92 percent slept restlessly.

Although pregnant women have always reported these sleep disturbances to their obstetricians/gynecologists (OB/GYNs), sleep researchers and clinicians have just recently focused their attention on sleep needs and changes in pregnancy. It is a challenge for researchers to study sleep changes in pregnancy. Obviously, to assess such hypothesized changes, researchers need to observe and evaluate women during each trimester, or even during each month of pregnancy. This is a rather daunting task for researchers. As a result, some studies have compared groups of women from each trimester of pregnancy (at various weeks within each trimester) to age-matched, nonpregnant controls. Other studies have focused on one particular trimester. Still others have followed the same women over the course of pregnancy. Unfortunately, because these study designs are so different, and because assessment techniques vary as well (e.g., sleep lab studies, self-report questionnaires, observations, and clinical interviews), it is difficult to draw conclusions. However, we certainly know far more than we used to about pregnancy and sleep, from the growing body of scientific and clinical literature as well as from women themselves.

Physiological and psychological changes during pregnancy and the early postpartum period affect a woman's sleep. Changes in hormones during the first trimester, the rapid growth of the fetus in the last trimester, and caring for a newborn with random sleep-wake patterns all may contribute to disrupted sleep. Yet, these disruptions and changes vary both from one woman to another and throughout pregnancy and in the postpartum months (Bassett, Giovanni, Peterson, McGurn, Trentacoste, Wolfson, and Anwer 1999; Lee 1998). In the National Sleep Foundation's Women and Sleep Poll (1998), 78 percent of the women polled stated that they experienced more disturbed sleep during pregnancy than they had at other times in their lives. During the first trimester, nausea, vomiting, backaches, and the increased need to urinate interrupts many women's sleep. In the second trimester, women may be awakened by fetal movements and heartburn; however, often their sleep improves at this point in pregnancy. Finally, during the third trimester, sleep is disrupted due to frequent urination, backaches, shortness of breath, and leg cramps. Some women also report that they experience more frequent frightening dreams and nightmares during pregnancy. In the sections below, I discuss the physiological changes that occur during pregnancy, and then review each trimester in greater detail. The diagram on the next page summarizes some of the key sleep changes during pregnancy.

Physiological Changes throughout Pregnancy

The normal gestation periods ranges from thirty-seven to forty-three weeks, with most births occurring between thirty-nine and forty-one weeks. During the first twelve weeks of pregnancy many hormonal changes take place, such as a rise in the secretion of estrogen, progesterone, and prolactin. In particular, progesterone is essential for the maintenance of pregnancy. Early in pregnancy, progesterone brings on drowsiness, rapid sleep onset, nausea, and frequent urination. Yet, some women experience difficulties falling asleep. The women's growing uterus begins to press on her bladder, and her breasts swell and become tender as milk glands develop.

During weeks thirteen through twenty-six, the second trimester, the growing baby begins to take up far more space and the woman's uterus begins to swell. By midpregnancy, the breasts become larger and heavier.

Changes in Sleep during Pregnancy

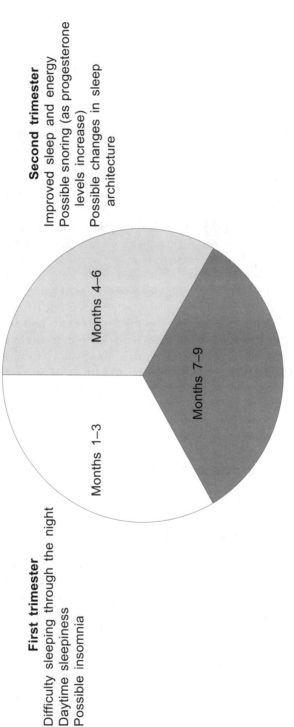

First trimester
Difficulty sleeping through the night
Daytime sleepiness
Possible insomnia

Second trimester
Improved sleep and energy
Possible snoring (as progesterone levels increase)
Possible changes in sleep architecture

Third trimester
Improved sleep and energy
Possible snoring (as progesterone levels increase)
Possible changes in sleep architecture

Months 1–3

Months 4–6

Months 7–9

In the third trimester, weeks twenty-seven through forty, the increasingly higher level of progesterone contributes to increased respiratory rates and shortness of breath. In addition, the enlarged uterus presses on the bladder, reducing capacity and increasing the need to urinate frequently. Due to the growing uterus, the diaphragm is restricted and breathing becomes shallower; the intestines and esophageal sphincter are displaced and softened, causing esophageal reflux and heartburn. The muscles in the uterus contract more and more often; these "practice" contractions are referred to as Braxton-Hicks contractions.

First Trimester (Months One through Three)

Although there are individual differences in women's pregnancies, many of you will find the first trimester to be the most tiring time of your pregnancy. You may find it difficult to sleep through the night and you may have considerable sleepiness throughout the day. As I mentioned earlier, sleep habits begin to change as early as the first trimester, particularly by weeks ten to twelve. During this period high levels of the natural hormone progesterone are produced, increasing sleepiness. As a result, during this time you may find yourself sleeping more than you did before you were pregnant, more even than you will later in pregnancy. The flood of progesterone may make an average day in the office seem as taxing as backpacking up a mountain; it may make you feel like you are coming down with a virus. Progesterone has also been shown to increase body temperature and to act on the smooth muscle of the urinary tract, causing frequent urination. You will find that your sleep is more disrupted as you wake up more and more to use the bathroom; your newly tender breasts may make it more difficult to find a comfortable sleeping position; and nausea can hit at any time during the day or night. A small number of women even experience insomnia in the first months of pregnancy. A friend and colleague talked with me at length about her pregnancy-related insomnia:

> I have a twenty-month old son and I am now sixteen weeks pregnant with my second child (a girl!). I tend to have problems sleeping in general when I am stressed out, but the first indication of serious sleep problems came when I was pregnant for the first time and I suffered from severe insomnia. At one point, I believe I went for ten days without sleep. I am not sure what to credit my sleep difficulties to. I have found with my second pregnancy that I have the same problem with insomnia. During the day, I can fall asleep at the drop of a hat, but if I do,

it makes the nights even more torturous. It seems that I can fall asleep fine, but inevitably, I wake up a few hours later . . . So, for the time being, I am resigned to it.

Second Trimester
(Months Four through Six)

Many of you will be relieved to move into the second trimester, when your sleep will improve at night and you may feel more energetic during the day. The second trimester is often referred to as the "honeymoon phase." Progesterone levels continue to rise, but more slowly than before. Also, the growing fetus places less pressure on the bladder since it now moves above it. As a result of both of these changes, many women will no longer need to urinate as frequently and, fortunately, experience better sleep during the second trimester than during the first. Some studies report changes in sleep architecture (e.g., to slow-wave sleep [SWS] and Rapid Eye Movement [REM] sleep) during the second trimester, but they are inconclusive at this time. Of course, you just might feel your baby move (called "quickening") for the first time while waiting to fall asleep.

In the second trimester, women may begin to snore for the first time in their lives. According to the National Sleep Foundation's Women and Sleep Poll (1998), about 30 percent of pregnant women report this new development. Snoring begins at this time because of increased swelling in women's nasal passages. This is apparently due to an increase in estrogen that may cause the capillaries of the nasal passages to swell and partially block airways.

Pregnant women who snore may be at risk of preeclampsia, also known as toxemia, and/or sleep apnea according to recent research. Health-care providers look for the following signs of preeclampsia in pregnant women: high blood pressure, swelling that doesn't go away, and large quantities of protein in the urine. Specifically, if the blockage of airways, caused by swelling from preeclampsia, is severe, sleep apnea may result, characterized by loud snoring and periods of stopped breathing during sleep (see chapter 8). The lack of oxygen that results from sleep apnea disrupts sleep and may affect the fetus. If you are told that you snore loudly, and you have severe daytime sleepiness (another symptom of sleep apnea and related disorders), please consult your health-care provider.

Third Trimester
(Months Seven through Nine)

Studies indicate that the quality of sleep in the last trimester is worse than during any other phase of pregnancy. In all likelihood, you will experience the most pregnancy-related sleep problems at this time, and you will probably feel physically uncomfortable. Heartburn, the need to urinate, leg cramps, and sinus congestion are common causes of disturbed sleep as you get closer to your due date. Many women also report increasing levels of morning fatigue over the course of the last trimester.

Leg cramps become quite common during pregnancy, especially during the third trimester. According to researchers, leg cramps are experienced by about 20 percent of women during the first trimester and 75 percent of women in the third trimester; fewer than 10 percent experience leg cramps at three months postpartum (Gupta, Schorck, and Gay 1992). Up to 20 percent of pregnant women develop Restless Legs Syndrome (RLS) during the third trimester. RLS symptoms are described as a feeling as if something is crawling or moving inside the foot, calf, and/or upper leg (Goodman, Brodie, and Ayida 1988). Recent research suggests that RLS during pregnancy may be due to decreased levels of iron (serum ferritin), or folate. If you have experienced leg cramps and/or RLS, you know that these symptoms disrupt your sleep throughout the night. Moving your leg can stop the symptoms temporarily, but the symptoms may return when your leg is still. Fortunately, for most women, the symptoms go away after the baby is born. However, women who are not pregnant can also suffer from RLS. If you experience leg cramps during or outside of pregnancy, it is highly recommended that you meet with your health-care provider to determine if the complaint is actually a more serious problem of RLS, or myoclonus (leg cramps) during sleep (see chapter 8). Unfortunately, medications customarily used to treat RLS may cause harm to the fetus, so you'll need to discuss their use with your health-care provider. Eating a nutritious diet may prevent abnormally low iron levels and other risks during pregnancy, thereby reducing the symptoms of RLS and leg cramps.

Overall, findings from studies indicate that pregnant women spend more time awake at night (reduced sleep efficiency) due to the many symptoms and physical changes that occur over the nine-month gestation period. In contrast, sleep architecture changes during pregnancy seem to be minimal. The amount of REM sleep either remains unchanged or diminishes only slightly. Research on changes in the amount of SWS during pregnancy remains inconclusive, but some studies document a reduction in slow-wave sleep (SWS) over the course of pregnancy. It appears that the more frequent and/or longer wakeful episodes during sleep have little effect on REM sleep, but they result in less SWS and decreased sleep efficiency (Lee 1998).

Historically, women have been told that disrupted sleep during pregnancy is their bodies' way of preparing for motherhood and future sleepless nights. However, you do not have to put up with these sleep difficulties. It is important for you to talk with your health-care provider if you experience significant changes in your sleep during pregnancy.

Sleep-Smart Strategies during Your Pregnancy

Prenatal care consists of three interrelated, but equally important, focal points: care for your self, care and support from friends and family members, and regular visits to a midwife or physician. Below are Sleep-Smart Strategies that you should include in your self-care throughout your pregnancy. Use these strategies to help alleviate sleep problems during pregnancy, either on your own or with the help of a sleep specialist.

* Sleep on your left side. During the third trimester, try to sleep on your left side, to allow for the best blood flow to the fetus and to your uterus and kidneys. Avoid lying flat on your back for long periods, since the increased pressure on your back and intestines can cause discomfort and make it difficult to sleep. You can place a pillow between your knees to help you sleep more comfortably on your side.

* Take naps. Naps may be beneficial. Research suggests that a planned thirty- to sixty-minute nap during the day can improve alertness and memory and can reduce symptoms of daytime sleepiness. It is noteworthy that in the National Sleep Foundation's Women and Sleep Poll (1998), just over 50 percent of pregnant women reported taking at least one weekday nap and 60 percent reported taking at least one weekend nap. (Note, however, that taking naps may not be advisable for people who experience insomnia.)

* Eat nutritious foods. Unquestionably, it is crucial to eat and drink well when you are pregnant. What you eat and drink can affect the quality of your sleep, particularly during pregnancy. Drink lots of fluids during the day, especially water. However, try to decrease your intake of fluids before bedtime so that you do not exacerbate your need to use the bathroom during the night. To prevent heartburn, avoid eating large amounts of spicy, acidic, or fried foods. You will find that it is also beneficial to eat several light meals throughout the day rather than a large meal close to bedtime. Foods high in protein and iron are recommended. Also,

if you experience nausea while you're trying to sleep, try frequent bland snacks (e.g., plain crackers) throughout the day.

* Exercise regularly. Regular activity will help you stay healthy, improve your circulation, and reduce leg cramps. It will help you sleep better. However, finish your vigorous exercise activities within three to four hours of bedtime. Working out too close to your bedtime may make it more difficult to fall asleep.

* Avoid nicotine and alcohol. Smoking and drinking during pregnancy can harm your baby. No safe limit has been established for alcohol consumption during pregnancy, and the consumption of as little as one to two ounces per day during the first trimester is associated with fetal alcohol syndrome (DiFranza and Lew 1995). Also, both substances can cause sleep difficulties, as I discussed in chapter 2. Moreover, smoking is associated with placenta abnormalities, miscarriage, premature delivery, and low birth weight. Infants born to mothers who smoke during pregnancy (approximately ten to fifty cigarettes per day) tend to be more difficult to rouse from sleep, are at risk for obstructive sleep apnea episodes, and may be more susceptible to sudden infant death syndrome (SIDS) (DiFranza and Lew 1995).

* Use treatment techniques to cope with insomnia symptoms. Insomnia is generally defined as the inability to fall asleep or maintain sleep. Many women experience insomnia symptoms during pregnancy. The following stimulus control techniques may be particularly helpful if you experience insomnia during pregnancy:

>   a. Try not to use your bed or bedroom for any activity other than sleep.
>
>   b. Establish a regular presleep routine.
>
>   c. When you get into bed, turn out the lights. If after ten to fifteen minutes you find that you're unable to sleep, get up and go to another room. Engage in a quiet activity until you feel drowsy, then return to your room to sleep
>
>   d. Repeat step *c* as often as necessary through the night, and use these same steps if you awaken during the night.

It is also important to follow these sleep hygiene tips:

>   a. Keep a fairly regular schedule for going to bed and waking up (your bedtime should be when you are drowsy).
>
>   b. Try to avoid naps.
>
>   c. Exercise regularly.
>
>   d. Get natural light exposure in the afternoon.

e. Avoid caffeine within six hours of bedtime.

f. Try to create a comfortable sleep environment.

g. Try not to worry about your sleep. (See chapter 7 for information on the symptoms and treatment of insomnia.)

Plan for the Future: Minimize Sleeplessness after Childbirth

The next chapter focuses on childbirth and the postpartum months. Yet, in all likelihood, throughout your pregnancy you have been contemplating and discussing with your partner a variety of child-rearing issues (e.g., Should my baby boy be circumcised? Will I nurse or bottle-feed? When will I go back to work?). I recommend you also discuss the issue of sleep (both yours and the baby's) at this point. While you are pregnant, you can plan where your baby will sleep, discuss what to do when he or she awakens during the night, and develop a bedtime ritual for your baby. In order to get an idea of what to expect after you bring your baby home, you may want to look at the Sleep-Smart Strategies for Your Baby, presented at the end of chapter 4. In a study that my colleagues and I conducted with first-time expectant parents, we found that expectant couples who learned how to promote healthy sleep patterns in their infants reported that they felt less stress and a greater sense of efficacy as parents, and that their infants woke up less often and slept longer than did parents who had not received such training (Wolfson, Lacks and Futterman 1992).

Fortunately or unfortunately, most of us (regardless of how good our sleep was before becoming mothers) experience some obvious changes in our sleep-wake patterns after we bring home our first child. One mother describes her experience this way:

> I had always been a good sleeper. Even when I was a child, my parents never had any problem getting me to go to bed. Throughout my twenties, I was also a good sleeper, usually falling asleep (if I had no social engagement) at around ten o'clock and waking without my alarm clock at the same time each morning, around half past six. I never had insomnia or trouble sleeping through the night. Most of the time, as soon as my head hit the pillow, I was asleep.
>
> When I became pregnant at the age of thirty-two, though, everything changed. When I was about five months pregnant, I would awake nearly every morning at around four o'clock and be unable to go back to sleep. I would usually get the

newspaper, which arrives early at my house, read it, and hopefully fall back asleep at around five. My friend had the same thing happen to her when she was pregnant and told me that it was "nature's way of preparing us for future night feedings."

Then, when my daughter was born, of course, all normal sleep patterns were thrown off. I nursed my baby for the first year. Until she was six months old, when she finally slept through the night, I would wake up at least once each night for a feeding. Now my daughter is an excellent sleeper, going to bed at seven o'clock and waking up between six and seven each morning. Yet I do not sleep as well as I used to. I usually have to read to get sleepy, and even though I am tired after putting my child to bed, I do not feel like sleeping. Those precious hours after seven o'clock are the few that I have to myself without having to take care of my daughter. As a result, I go to bed later than I probably should. And even when I sleep, I still feel like I am on call, waking up and automatically worrying about my daughter. Furthermore, unlike my pre-motherhood years, instead of waking up on my own before the alarm clock, I wake up when I hear my daughter calling for me. My daughter is my wake-up call, putting me on duty as soon as she wakes up.

* 4 *

Childbirth and Postpartum Months: Sleeping for Two or More

Historically, research on women's sleep after childbirth focused on infants' sleep-wake patterns. Yet, obviously, your sleep is changed or even transformed once your baby is born, independent of your baby's sleep patterns. In this chapter, I will discuss labor and delivery, the postpartum months (during which mood and sleep are intricately entwined), as well as strategies to help you plan for better sleep when your baby arrives.

Most women find that they are tired from poor sleep during their third trimester (not to mention the entire pregnancy) as they head into labor. The experience of labor and delivery is hard on the body and women in labor are kept awake during the night struggling with contractions (I was up all night with painful contractions due to back labor when my son was born). A tiny new person to care for day and night and the realization that one's life is now changed from what it once was—no wonder we are all so tired!

The Postpartum Experience

Clearly, your sleep quality diminishes as you approach labor and begin those early weeks of motherhood. In our study of 41 pregnant mothers, the women were particularly bothered by not being able to find a comfortable position to sleep, waking up frequently to use the bathroom, feeling too hot or perspiring, and feeling their babies' movements (Wolfson and Anwer 2000). However, research has not shown a relationship between sleep quality and quantity and any perinatal adverse outcome, length of labor, or type of delivery

(Evans, Dick, and Clark 1995). For the most part, sleep efficiency and quality are lousy on a woman's first night after delivery, but sleep begins to improve over the following days and weeks.

The postpartum period is generally defined as the first six months after delivery, but some experts define it as lasting from lactation to when the infant is sleeping through the night with predictable day-night sleeping patterns. This remarkable period begins with the birth of the infant and the release of the hormone-secreting placenta. In the early postpartum days there is a rapid fall in placental hormones; as a result 35 to 80 percent of women experience postpartum distress, or "baby blues," approximately three to five days after birth. During these blues or mood swings, many women feel happy one minute and sad the next. Many feel a little depressed and have a hard time concentrating. For women, the blues are confined to the first week following childbirth, but for approximately 10 to 15 percent of new mothers, the blues continue and develop into postpartum depression closer to two to four weeks postpartum (O'Hara 1987; Rollins 1996). Some of the symptoms of postpartum depression are:

* loss of interest or pleasure in formerly enjoyable activities
* loss of appetite
* decreased energy and motivation
* difficulty falling and/or staying asleep
* sleeping more than usual
* increased crying or tearfulness
* feeling worthless, hopeless, or overly guilty
* feeling restless, irritable, or anxious
* unexplained weight loss or gain
* feeling like life is not worth living
* having thoughts about hurting yourself
* worrying about hurting your baby

If you experience symptoms of postpartum depression, you are strongly advised to seek professional help from your physician, a psychologist, psychiatrist, or other mental health practitioner. Postpartum depression is treated with therapy, support networks, and medications, such as antidepressants. In addition to seeking professional help, mothers with postpartum depression may find it constructive and beneficial to

* talk to someone about your feelings and thoughts;
* make use of friends, family members, and/or hired help who can assist you with child care, household chores, and errands;

* make time to do something for yourself each day, even for only fifteen minutes (e.g., reading, exercising, walking, taking a bath, or meditating;

* keep a diary—write down your emotions or thoughts, and then write down a more positive way of looking at or thinking about that emotion or thought;

* keep your expectations simple; for example, allow yourself to get only one thing done each day;

* give yourself permission to feel overwhelmed by your new role as mother;

* find a support group in your area.

Studies suggest that postpartum depression is more likely to occur if you have experienced previous postpartum depression, depression prior and unrelated to your pregnancy, severe symptoms related to premenstrual syndrome (PMS), and/or a stressful life event during pregnancy or after childbirth. The cause of postpartum depression is not known. Although progesterone and estrogen levels decrease during the first few postpartum days, information on the relationship between hormone levels and postpartum depression or mood changes are inconclusive, at best.

Psychologists argue that our culture expects new mothers to be depressed, and that modern society encourages women to label emotions and bodily sensations (perhaps due to hormone fluctuations) experienced in the postpartum months as "baby blues" (Unger and Crawford 1992). Simply labeling these feelings as baby blues does not take into account many other aspects of the social situation of the new mother (and father), such as the level of social support, the health of the baby, the type of delivery and the level of difficulty of the labor, and other contextual variables. One additional contextual factor in postpartum depression that seems obvious to this author and to many mothers, but that has been overlooked by researchers and clinicians, is sleep deprivation and other sleep-wake changes. In the 1990s, researchers finally began to assess sleep deprivation as a variable in postpartum mood changes (Lee, McEnany, and Zaffke 2000; Wilkie and Shapiro 1992; Wolfson and Anwer 2000). In the next few section, I describe and refer to some of the findings from these noteworthy studies.

Mothers' Sleep-Wake Patterns after Childbirth

I often chuckle to myself when I think about sleep researchers, like myself, hypothesizing that women's sleep changes in the early postpartum days and weeks. You do not have to do a scientific study to conclude that sleep is disrupted following childbirth and, perhaps, throughout parenthood. One such study found that nearly 30 percent of new mothers' sleep was disturbed because of their babies' sleep-wake schedules, the new responsibilities of parenthood, and discomfort from breastfeeding, etc. (Salzarulo 1987). One friend and colleague of mine recalled:

> During pregnancy I often had trouble sleeping because I woke up three or four times a night to go to the bathroom. When my children were born, I usually slept for only about three to four hours uninterrupted. Then I would have to get up to nurse the baby. After that, I would only get a few more hours to rest before I had to get up in the morning. Our sleep schedules were typically opposite. My newborn's day was my night, while my day was my baby's night. Therefore, I would typically try to nap when my baby napped, but that rarely worked, and I felt exhausted during the day.

Another friend commented:

> I was exhausted after I had my first child, a baby boy—in fact, I had never been so tired in my life. I felt that it was a cumulative process. During the first week the baby was home, I was up a lot. Six months later, with this still going on, I was a mess. I had another child two years after my first. I was exhausted from my second pregnancy and then I had a baby and a two-year-old toddler to take care of, not to mention going back to work.

In my own research, my colleagues and I assessed, through daily sleep diaries, forty-one first-time mothers' sleep and mood from the last four weeks of pregnancy through twelve months postpartum. These women reported that their sleep efficiency (i.e., minutes actually asleep relative to their time in bed) in the first two to four postpartum weeks was significantly lower than it had been during the end of their last trimester. These first-time mothers reported an average of one hour of awake time each night at the end of their pregnancies in comparison to over two hours in those early postpartum weeks. Obviously, their sleep was disrupted due to their babies' night wakings. Yet, by four months postpartum, their sleep efficiency had returned to its last trimester level. Other researchers report that women experience a decline in sleep efficiency from the third trimester to the first postpartum month (Waters and Lee 1996). In my research team's study of first-time mothers, the number of minutes of disruptions continued to decrease over the remainder of the first year postpartum (four to twelve months). It is unclear whether women's sleep patterns return to normal by the baby's first birthday; however, in reviewing my preliminary data, it certainly looks like there is considerable improvement in sleep efficiency at twelve months over the first month after the baby is born. Also, the women reported more napping in the early postpartum months, but more sleep complaints (e.g., physical discomfort, need to urinate during the night, or thoughts running through their mind) and diminished sleep quality in the final weeks before delivery (Evans, Dick, and Clark 1995; Wolfson and Anwer 2000). As women themselves have known for years, sleep is terribly disrupted both during pregnancy as well as throughout the postpartum months.

Some women find that their sleep is more disrupted following the birth of their first child than following the birth of their second and third children. Sleep researchers Morning Waters and Kathryn Lee (1996) found this to be true in their laboratory study that compared first-time mothers to second- and third-time mothers in their sleep disturbances, fatigue, and daytime functioning. Studies have also shown that mothers, regardless of the number of children, have a significant increase in slow-wave sleep (SWS) and a decrease in Stages 1 and 2 or light sleep at one month postpartum (Driver and Shapiro 1992; Waters and Lee 1996). Whether this is your first or fourth child, if your baby is waking you up several times each night while your body is simultaneously adjusting to its post-pregnancy (and possible lactating) state, you're bound to feel pretty tired and out of balance during the day.

Sleep and Mood in the Postpartum Months

Obviously, considerable sleep-wake pattern changes take place during pregnancy and after childbirth, yet little is known about how these changes affect women's mental health during and after pregnancy. Previous postpartum mood literature largely concentrated on variables such as social support, work activities, socioeconomic status, age, and general physical health as factors leading to postpartum depression. Not surprising to most women, recent studies have documented a strong relationship between sleep and mood from pregnancy through the first three to four postpartum months (Lee, McEnany, and Zaffke 2000). Certainly sleep deprivation would make it difficult for most of us to feel chipper, upbeat, and energetic enough to change diapers every hour, nurse nonstop, and host all of our relatives and friends. Yet only recently have sleep researchers and clinicians begun to understand the complex relationship between sleep and mood during this time and been able to provide recommendations to women, going through these life changes.

Specifically, Grant Wilkie and Colin Shapiro (1992) found that nighttime labor and a history of sleep disruption at the end of pregnancy were related to a higher incidence of postpartum blues. In our study in which we followed more than forty-one women from the last trimester of pregnancy through twelve months postpartum, sleep problems were associated with depressed mood within periods of a few weeks. In particular, increased sleep complaints (e.g., physical discomfort or thoughts running through the woman's mind during the night), increased time spent awake due to disruptions, and decreased total sleep were most associated with reports of depressed mood (Wolfson and Anwer 2000).

Sleep-wake patterns were also related to depressed mood later on. For example, increased time spent awake due to disruptions at the end of pregnancy and at two to three weeks postpartum were linked to higher levels of depressed mood at approximately four months. And increased time spent awake due to disruptions at approximately four months postpartum was associated with increased depressed mood at twelve months after their babies were born. It appears that critical sleep disruption during pregnancy and just after childbirth may cause some women to be more vulnerable to experiencing depressed mood or emotional instability particularly in the early postpartum weeks or months.

Furthermore, Rapid Eye Movement (REM) sleep probably has an important influence on mood and thought. Kathryn Lee and colleagues (2000) assessed REM sleep during pregnancy at each trimester and at one month postpartum in more than thirty women. REM latency (length of time before first REM episode) was highly variable during pregnancy, but the quantity of REM sleep was very stable across the three trimesters of pregnancy. Mood state was also stable during the women's pregnancies; the most negative moods were reported during three to four weeks postpartum, findings that are similar to those of our study. Although progesterone decreases from the third trimester to the postpartum period, total REM sleep did not seem to change over this period. However, Lee found that REM latency decreased significantly from the last trimester to three to four weeks postpartum. REM latencies were significantly shorter (under one hour) for the postpartum women with self-reported higher levels of depressed mood.

Most women expect to deal with interrupted sleep once their baby is born and during those early years of motherhood. However, if you experience considerable sleep disruption and negative mood during pregnancy and in the early postpartum months, it will be helpful for you to strategize in advance as to how to prepare yourself and your family for the difficult times ahead. See Sleep-Smart Strategies for Mother (and Fathers) for recommendations for taking care of yourself as you enter parenthood. For now, let's switch gears and learn about infants' sleep-wake patterns.

Parenting Practices and Babies' Sleep-Wake Patterns

Your baby's developing sleep patterns certainly affect your own sleep-wake schedule and vice versa. In this section, I discuss the complex interactions that take place between parents and infants with regard to sleep in the early months and years.

Disrupted sleep is generally accepted as an inevitable part of life with young babies. At Lamaze class reunions, family gatherings, daycare interviews, and so on, parents of newborns are often asked, "Is your baby sleeping through the night?" "How much sleep did you get last night?" However, parenting classes and books often do not focus on preventing sleep problems. Instead they focus on other worthwhile subjects, such as labor and delivery, breastfeeding, car-seat use, early developmental milestones, and safe baby toys. Pediatricians, early childhood educators, child psychologists, and others are unlikely to systematically assist parents with their infants' sleep-wake habits much less the parents' own sleep needs.

Consequently, parent surveys show that early, stable sleeping patterns are often not established; 20 to 30 percent of young children have trouble falling asleep and staying asleep during their first three to four years (Lozoff, Wolf, and Davis 1985; Zuckerman, Stevenson, and Bailey 1987). Moreover, at least 5 percent of mothers of young infants report that their own sleep is disrupted by their baby (Zuckerman, Stevenson, and Bailey 1987). Clearly, sleeping difficulties are common among babies and young children and may affect the sleep and daytime functioning of their mothers (and fathers).

The expression "sleeping through the night" is misleading because most of us, children and adults, periodically wake up at various times throughout the night. For the most part, however, we fall right back to sleep and do not recall these brief awakenings the next morning. Over the years, studies have shown that even when parents claim that their baby sleeps through the night, time-lapse video of the babies has demonstrated that only one-sixth of two-month-olds and one-third of nine-month-olds seem to sleep through the night (Anders and Keener 1985). Likewise, in Dr. Isabel Paret's study of nine-month-olds, all of the babies woke up at least once during the night, and many of the babies fell back to sleep without the parents knowing they had awakened (Paret 1983).

My advice, and the advice of other researchers (Cuthbertson and Schevill 1985), then, is not to expect your two- to nine-month-old child to sleep for an uninterrupted eight, ten, or twelve hours. Instead, you can begin to help your baby or toddler to become independent during the night and not require mother's or father's assistance to fall back to sleep upon awakening.

Over the course of the first year and thereafter, unintentional habits may develop when older infants and toddlers establish an association between their parent's presence and their ability to fall asleep. As a result, when the infant awakens, she feels that she needs her mother or father to be present in order to fall back to sleep. In fact, infants whose parents are present, perhaps rubbing the baby's back, when they fall asleep at bedtime are significantly more likely to wake up at night than infants whose parents do not remain in the room until they fall sound asleep (Adair, Bauchner, Philipp, Levenson, and Zuckerman 1991; France, Henderson, and Hudson 1996). Repeated associations between the baby's crying, the parent's attention, and the baby's resumption of sleep sometimes make it difficult for babies to begin to soothe themselves, experience fewer lengthy awakenings, and fall back to sleep on their own. See Sleep-Smart Strategies for Your Baby, later in this chapter, for tips on establishing good sleep habits for your child.

As emphasized above, how a child falls asleep and how his parents interact with him with regard to his sleep are crucial aspects of sleep-wake development. Sleeping arrangements may also affect the developing sleep-wake patterns in children. The relationship between sleeping arrangements (e.g., co-sleeping, sleeping alone, or sharing bedroom with sibling) and sleep disruptions is poorly understood. Until recently, nearly all studies of infant sleep organization and development have been conducted on infants sleeping alone. Likewise, over the years pediatric and psychology professionals in the United States have recommended that children sleep alone. Even so, some degree of co-sleeping (meaning the parents and child sleep together in the same bed) is reported in about half of the families with young children in the United States (Lozoff 1995). Whether and when families choose to co-sleep, differs between families and across cultural groups. Some families immediately begin co-sleeping with their newborn, whereas others decide to bring the baby into the parents' bed when the baby wakes up at night and has trouble going back to sleep.

Recent research has found that mothers and infants who co-sleep may wake up more often and spend more time awake during the night than they do when sleeping alone (McKenna, Thomas, Anders, Sadeh, Schechtman, and Glotzbach 1993). Certainly more research needs to be done to completely determine the effects of co-sleeping. It appears that co-sleeping on an ongoing basis may not be a good idea if you and your baby want a good night's sleep; however, co-sleeping works for some families and not for others, so you should use your own judgment when deciding whether to co-sleep and see what works best for you.

Infant feeding also is a central concern of many mothers, especially first-time breastfeeding mothers. Anecdotal reports from clinicians working with breastfeeding mothers indicate that fatigued mothers tend to have difficulty breastfeeding. Although there are many hypotheses regarding sleep (infants and mothers) and mothers' feeding practices, it remains unclear whether there are any recognizable differences in sleep between mothers who bottle feed and those who breastfeed. In our study, mothers who primarily bottle fed did not report different sleep patterns from those of mothers who breastfed in the first four months. One researcher assessed the sleeping patterns of breastfeeding mothers versus bottle-feeding mothers. The results showed that the breastfeeding mothers reported more night wakings than the bottle-feeding mothers, but there were no differences in total hours of sleep between the groups (Quillen 1997). So if you choose to breastfeed, you can probably expect to be awakened during the night to nurse, but you and your baby will also benefit physically and emotionally from breastfeeding. Contact a lactation expert if you have any problems breastfeeding.

Given the many influences on children's sleep, child and infant sleep patterns are quite variable. Many of the factors, such as maturation and medical problems, are not easy or possible to control. Parenting practices regarding child sleep, however, may be altered to encourage healthy sleep-wake patterns in infants, children, and their parents. Both child and parent influence and shape the other's responses. Parenting style varies from family to family, yet certain practices tend to be more beneficial to your baby's developing sleep/wake habits than others. For example, you may find that when you and/or your partner are inconsistent and anxious, your child's sleep becomes more problematic and disordered (Crowell, Keener, Ginsburg, and Anders 1987). Undoubtedly, picking the child up, rocking him or her to sleep, and feeding an older baby in the middle of the night seem to increase night wakings and an inability to fall asleep without help. However, parents can increase their knowledge about infant sleep and learn to respond to their child in a way that will promote good, healthy sleep patterns early on for the entire family (Adair, Zuckerman, Bauchner, Philipp, and Levenson 1992; Wolfson, Lacks, and Futterman 1992).

Pediatricians, psychologists, journalists, and parents have written books and designed parenting programs to help parents to develop healthy sleep habits in their child (Cuthbertson and Schevill

1985; Ferber 1985; Mindell 1997; Weissbluth 1987). These books and programs provide information for parents about how to promote good sleep habits in their children early on. Although intervention procedures are available for treating sleep disturbances in children, it is critical to try to prevent such problems in the first place.

Parents who have realistic expectations about parenthood feel more competent and less stressed about how to respond to their child's sleeping behaviors (Durand and Mindell 1990; Wolfson, Lacks, and Futterman 1992). The birth of a child and the outset of parenthood is a stressful time. Although birth is usually viewed as a positive experience, many of the associated life changes are frequently perceived as negative or stressful (e.g., less time for self/spouse, changes in sleep patterns). In families where the infant is not sleeping through the night, parents are often sleep deprived, less alert during the day, and therefore highly frazzled and stressed (Durand and Mindell 1990; Wolfson, Lacks, and Futterman 1992). Furthermore, infant and toddler night wakings and other sleep disturbances may lead to increased family arguments regarding the best solution (Durand and Mindell 1993), decreased family satisfaction (Scott and Richards 1990), and less-confident parenting (Wolfson, Lacks, and Futterman 1992).

Sleep-Smart Strategies for Mothers

Below are strategies for you (as well as for your spouse or partner) to try in order to decrease exhaustion in the early postpartum weeks and months and so that you feel more competent, less hassled, and more equipped to guide your baby toward developing good sleep habits early on.

* Have sensible expectations. All of us imagine ourselves swaying back and forth in our grandmother's rocking chair, singing and rocking our baby to sleep. But you won't need to rock your baby to sleep every night until she enters kindergarten, or rub your son's back every night until he starts junior high. Know that you can help your baby learn healthy sleep habits, but don't expect her to sleep "through the night" right away. Over the course of the first year, as her need for night feedings decreases and she settles into her daily and nightly routines, you can gradually help her to learn to soothe herself and become more independent during the night. Know also that your sleep is very important, too. It is crucial that mothers (and fathers) obtain adequate sleep for themselves so that we may be alert, focused, and able to enjoy

our children during the daytime. Don't expect yourself to function normally and feel good when you haven't had enough sleep.

✳ Study baby-sleep strategies in advance. It is far easier to be proactive and to teach your baby (and yourself) healthy sleep habits early on. Taking a preventive approach will reduce the likelihood that you or your child will develop sleep problems in the future. Therefore, read about infants' sleep, and determine your family's sleep rules before your baby is born, because once the baby arrives you will be sleep deprived and exhausted, making it difficult to make rational, well-thought-out plans.

✳ Work with your partner. If you are married or co-parenting, work together and prioritize your sleep as well as your baby's. Many of us forget that we need sleep, too! Here's the schedule that my husband and I began when our son, Noah, was about two weeks old (he's now nine years old): I would pump a bottle of breast milk between nine and ten o'clock at night and then go to sleep. My husband would wake Noah and feed him between ten and eleven o'clock and then put him back in his crib. If Noah awakened later, say at two in the morning, I'd nurse him. That way both my husband and I got at least five or six hours of sleep each night.

✳ Sleep when your baby sleeps. Simply put, in the early postpartum weeks, it is crucial that you try to sleep when your baby is sleeping rather than using that time to do household chores or catch up on work. When your baby naps, try to nap as well.

✳ Seek social support. Research suggests that social support (from dependable, loving friends or family members) may help prevent or diminish the stresses that many first-time mothers experience. However, you may find it best to limit the number of visitors in the early postpartum weeks. In my own study of mothers from the last trimester through twelve months postpartum (Wolfson and Anwer 2000), women who had too many visitors in the early postpartum weeks reported that they did not have time to nap and rest. There are several different types of social support: emotional support (e.g., listening to the new mother's feelings), social network support (assistance from family, friends, colleagues, etc.), tangible support (actually doing some sort of task for the mother such as baby-sitting so that she can run errands or rest), and informational support (providing information to the mother, such as an article on infant sleep). Some of you will find one type of social support more helpful than others depending on the situation and your needs at the time. Tangible social support (people you can depend on to help with actual tasks) is often advantageous with regard to sleep. You are likely to find that those friends, family members, and/or child-care providers who help take care of your new baby, giving you time to actually sleep, are most beneficial in those early postpartum weeks and months.

Sleep-Smart Strategies for Your Baby

First of all, there are two valuable principles that I swear by with regard to children's sleep issues: (1) parents are the ones in control of their infant's sleep and feeding, not the infant; and (2) parents need to foster independence in their infant and competence in themselves. Below are Sleep-Smart Strategies that will be beneficial to both you and your baby in the early postpartum months.

* Understand your child's sleep patterns and have age-appropriate expectations. During these early months newborns' needs are simple, yet seemingly unrelenting; you may feel exhausted during these early weeks. Remember that newborns' sleeping patterns center around the stomach; at first they sleep most of the time, waking up when they're hungry and falling asleep after eating. Gradually this pattern changes: newborns who want to eat ten times a day may be satisfied with only five larger feedings when they reach about three months of age. As the weeks go by, babies spend more time awake during the day, with their naps becoming more regular, and their sleep at night becomes more consolidated. The first four months of life are not a period of major physical milestones, but of laying neurological groundwork and forming an environment for future achievements.

* Develop and practice bedtime rituals and routines. Infants, like adults, benefit from a regular schedule. A routine provides an infant with security amid the many changes in her life. Variations in individual sleep needs are large, but everyone is better off having about the same amount of sleep, at about the same time each day. The more regular and predictable a young child's sleep routine is, the more flexible parents can be, without negative effects, when exceptions arise. Early on, at your baby's bedtime when he or she is sleepy, try a soothing activity such as song or story, place the baby in the crib and encourage him or her to cuddle with a transitional object (stuffed animal, or other soft toy), then say good night and leave the room while he or she is still awake. Repeat your routine every night at bedtime. My husband and I have been singing the same bedtime songs to our son since he

was just a few months old. He still loves the routine and recently told me that he'll sing them to himself when he is at overnight camp this summer.

* Teach your child to fall asleep on her own. Try not to hold, rock, or nurse your baby while she falls asleep. It's best not to teach your baby to rely on you to help her fall asleep. Since building a close relationship is important in those early weeks, hold your baby during her wakeful times rather than sleepy times. When your baby calls or cries out to you from her crib, I recommend that you or your partner return to reassure her and then leave again; gradually lengthen the time before responding to your fussing child until she self-soothes and falls asleep on her own. Understand that the phrase "sleeping through the night" refers *not* to an uninterrupted eight to twelve hours of sleep. Rather, "sleeping through the night" happens when the infant self-soothes and falls back to sleep on her own when she wakes up.

* Help your child to go back to sleep when he wakes during the night. During the first two to three months, your baby may need to be fed once or twice during the night. When your infant reaches eight weeks of age, is gaining weight continuously, and weighs at least nine to ten pounds (Wolfson, Lacks and Futterman 1992), you are encouraged to gradually move the late-night feeding to a later time, to lengthen the time before removing your fussing baby from the crib, to stretch the time between middle-of-the-night feedings, and to get your baby to settle until early morning without another feeding. After the age of two to three months, babies may continue to wake up during the night even at times when they do not need to be fed or changed. If your baby, toddler or young child wakes for reasons you cannot determine, she may be developing a pattern of night waking. If this is the case, it is recommended that you respond to night wakings as you do at bedtime, waiting increasingly longer between visits until your child soothes himself back to sleep. It is crucial to gradually stretch the time before responding in order to teach your child to self-soothe and go back to sleep without parental assistance.

* Offer rewards. Families may find it helpful to reward older toddlers and preschoolers in the morning for having fallen back to sleep on their own (e.g., with stickers).

* Keep a sleep-wake diary. Recording your child's progress in a sleep-wake diary can help your family adhere to a routine that increases the quality and quantity of both your sleep and your child's sleep.

* 5 *

Sleep-Wake Patterns during Menopause

While I was preparing to write this chapter, a colleague shared her experience with me, which you may find rather familiar:

> I experienced changes in my sleep during menopause, which lasted about three or four years. Hot flashes would disrupt my sleep nearly every night. During a hot flash, I'd become very warm, begin to sweat profusely, and feel irritated. I'd wake up throwing the covers off of my body. Some hot flashes were more intense than others were and they were sporadic at times. And I'd have eight to ten of these hot flashes a night, on average. Sometimes it seemed like I would just be falling into a deep sleep and then I would be awakened by a hot flash. This cycle of almost falling into a deep sleep and then being woken by another hot flash repeated itself many times during the night. In the morning, I would not be drowsy, just exhausted. At first, I did not pay much attention to the hot flashes. It took some time to realize exactly what was going on and why I felt so tired and run-down all the time. I did not connect it to the hot flashes immediately because I was only half awake when they occurred and not completely conscious of them. It is different from when your children wake you up during the night. In the morning, you remember that you got up to take care of them, but you do not remember the hot flashes so vividly. I was very grateful that I had a good amount of flexibility in my job; sometimes I was even able to return home for lunch and take a nap. Now I experience fewer hot flashes and they are more spaced out. Now that the hot flashes have abated, I am not tired all of the time and have plenty of energy.

Obviously, sleep disruption can affect how we feel both physically and emotionally. Researchers and clinicians have documented that both men's and women's sleep becomes more disrupted with advancing age. However, as we age, sleep patterns vary between men and women (Mauri 1990). Women report higher rates of sleep disturbance than men at all ages. In particular, women experience an increase in sleep disturbances during their midlife years, just before and during menopause. In this chapter, I define perimenopause and menopause, discuss some of the sleep changes that occur during this time in your life, present information regarding hormone replacement therapy (HRT) and its relationship to sleep-wake patterns, and, finally, provide recommendations for improving your sleep during perimenopause and menopause.

Understanding Menopause and Perimenopause

Many of you may have ideas of what menopause is all about as a result of what you've read, heard from your own mothers or grandmothers, and seen depicted in the media. Negative stereotypes have dominated most people's views of menopause for many years. Thankfully, we now have healthier perspectives and greater knowledge regarding menopause. In fact, during menopause many women feel more self-confident and view this period in their lives as a time of emotional and spiritual transformation.

So, what exactly is menopause? *Menopause* means the conclusion of menstruation, usually confirmed when a woman has not had a menstrual period for twelve consecutive months, in the absence of any other obvious cause. Menopause is a biological event—the end of fertility—resulting from the ovaries' decreased production of the sex hormones estrogen and progesterone. Menopause happens to all women, but it affects each woman uniquely.

Currently approximately 40 to 50 million women (more than one-third of American women) are estimated to be menopausal (*Our Bodies, Ourselves* 1998). A majority of women experience "natural menopause" (not caused by any medical intervention) between the ages of forty-five and fifty-five, on average at about age fifty-one. Some women experience menopause earlier (in their forties or even thirties), and a few go through it in their sixties. Women often experience menopause around the same age as their female relatives (e.g., mothers, sisters, and aunts) have. Others come to the post-menopausal stage following some sort of medical intervention, such as surgical removal of both ovaries, radiation treatments, chemotherapy, or use of certain drugs. It is important to note that a hysterectomy (surgical removal of the uterus) does not induce menopause if the ovaries are not removed.

I have found that there is considerable confusion regarding when menopause really takes place because many of the discomforts and difficulties such as menstrual irregularities, severe PMS, and sometimes hot flashes occur during the years leading up to menopause, the perimenopausal period. *Perimenopause*, which literally means "around menopause," refers to the menopause transition—the four- to eight-year period immediately prior to menopause when the changes of menopause begin. You should know that until you have completed the process of menopause (having had no periods for one year), you could still become pregnant. If you do not smoke, low dose oral contraceptives can be used right up until menstrual periods cease altogether.

Approximately 80 percent of women experience menopausal symptoms—hot flashes, night sweats, and vaginal dryness (Domar and Dreher 1996). Declining estrogen levels during menopause are frequently accompanied by hot flashes (unexpected feelings of heat and sweatiness throughout the body), and feelings of discomfort. Depressed mood, increased irritability, and insomnia are also frequently associated with menopause. Less common symptoms include headaches, weight gain, dizziness, and unfocused thinking. It is important to note that researchers have no definitive understanding of the relationship between hormone changes, mood, and sleep. Nonetheless, several studies have pointed out that perimenopausal women experience longer and more frequent awakenings from sleep than premenopausal women do. And sleep and mood changes are highly associated for perimenopausal women.

As Alice Domar, Ph.D., and Henry Dreher (1996) emphasize in their book, *Healing Mind, Healthy Woman*, I cannot state strongly enough that most women do not suffer or become invalids during the transition into menopause. This stereotypical view of menopause resulted from the opinions of physicians, researchers, and other health-care practitioners (largely men) who met with small, self-selected populations of women with menopausal symptoms. In fact, the majority of women do not even consult their doctors during their natural transition into menopause.

Premenopausal women who experience induced menopause do not go through the perimenopause transition; instead they must adjust to immediate menopause and the changes it brings. Such an abrupt loss of estrogen may cause severe menopause-related disturbances such as hot flashes. Furthermore, research suggests that women with induced menopause may be at greater risk for health problems such as heart disease and osteoporosis since they spend more years without the protective effects of estrogen.

In recent years, many physicians, psychologists, nurses, and other experts in women's health have written about the challenges, and the feelings of excitement and personal power, that accompany the menopausal years. But even through menopausal symptoms disrupt the sleep of many women, sleep challenges are not discussed in most of these books. In the National Sleep Foundation's Women and Sleep Poll (1998), 36 percent of menopausal women reported hot flashes during sleep. On average, they occurred three days each week and interfered with sleep five days per month. Moreover, as my colleague described at the beginning of this chapter, because hot flashes interrupt sleep and cause frequent wakings, they therefore contribute to significant daytime sleepiness. Understanding how your sleep is affected during menopause may help you to cope with its challenges. So let's examine menopause as it relates to sleep.

Menopausal Years and Sleep

As women get older, the amount of deep sleep (Stages 3 and 4) decreases, sleep becomes lighter, and more and longer awakenings occur during the night. Disturbed sleep is the most common complaint that brings women to menopause clinics. For example, 65 percent of women who visit the Yale Mid-Life Center experience insomnia (Keefe, Watson, and Naftolin 1999). Insomnia, restlessness, and lethargy are common complaints for menopausal women. In general, women report increased sleep disturbances, such as night wakings, in and around the menopausal years (Owens and Mathews 1998). Specifically, women who experience hot flashes find that their sleep is particularly less efficient than that of women who are not bothered by such hot flashes (Shaver, Giblin, Lentz, and Lee 1988).

Hot Flashes

Here is one woman's description of her experience with hot flashes:

> My fever broke. I woke at four o'clock in the morning and the bed was soaked. My whole body was perspiring. I said to myself, "Well, it is good that the fever has broken. What fever? I didn't know I had a fever. Well, I feel fine now. If I could just get back to sleep. I don't seem tired anymore. But I need more sleep. Surely I can fall asleep soon." In the next four hours, I changed my position an endless number of times. I tried to clear my mind. I thought good thoughts. I just couldn't sleep. When the same thing happened several times in the next few

weeks, I consulted my physician. I was told that the "night sweats" constituted an early symptom of menopause. Ever since then, experiencing these uncomfortable temperature changes in the middle of the night has made my life difficult. The insomnia associated with menopause has been my most obvious and troublesome symptom of midlife. I think that I will be able to cope with menopause as long as I can find a way to sleep again.

Hot flashes are the sign most commonly associated with menopause. Surveys report that approximately 50 to 85 percent of women experience hot flashes over a period of about five years, although some women do not find them irritating (Kronenberg 1990). During a hot flash, many women have a sudden increase in heart rate, or palpitations, an increase in peripheral blood flow that leads to a rise in skin temperature and causes perspiration. When the sweat evaporates, the body cools down and the woman may feel chilled (similar to having a mild fever).

According to circadian-rhythms researchers, hot flashes follow a daily cycle, peaking for most women in the late evening, when body temperature is highest. For other women, they peak in the morning, when body temperature is at its lowest point. Yet, as you may know from personal experience, hot flashes are usually most disturbing at night when they disrupt your sleep. Although they usually last only a few minutes, a few women experience severe hot flashes that wake them up about one hundred times each night. When nighttime hot flashes are particularly severe, they are referred to as *night sweats*. Friends have told me that on some nights they have perspired so much that they have had to get up and change their sheets and nightclothes. The loss of sleep is probably far more disruptive than the hot flashes themselves. Inefficient sleep as a result of hot flashes or night sweats may cause excessive daytime sleepiness, irritability, anxiety, and depressed mood. Some women find that sleep problems continue after their hot flashes have diminished. One of the prominent researchers in this area, Suzanne Woodward (1994) found that a menopausal woman's sleep is disrupted by brief awakenings every eight minutes if she is experiencing hot flashes, in comparison to every eighteen minutes if she is not. Woodward points out that in addition to awakenings from sleep, the changing temperatures associated with hot flashes can increase the amount of one of the sleep stages, slow-wave sleep (SWS). Treatment (e.g., HRT, relaxation techniques, or behavioral interventions) can reduce or eliminate hot flashes, improve sleep, improve daytime functioning, and prevent frequent night wakings from continuing after hot flashes subside. At the end of this chapter, some of these techniques are presented.

Then again, other sleep experts (Clark, Flowers, Boots, and Shettar 1995) suggest that hot-flash activity is not the main factor in midlife women's sleep-wake patterns. In other words, it is not clear whether sleep disturbances and/or changes across the perimeno-pausal/menopausal years are related to hormone changes versus the aging process. Without a doubt, hot flashes are terribly disruptive to sleep at this point in a women's lives.

Insomnia

A relatively common complaint of perimenopausal women is insomnia or sleeplessness. Insomnia means having trouble falling asleep, difficulty staying asleep, and/or the feeling that your sleep was not adequate for you. As discussed earlier, some women experience hot flashes at night, when their sleep is interrupted by frequent wakings and as a result is not refreshing or restorative. For the most part, once the hot flashes or night sweats have dissipated, women return to their normal sleep pattern. However, some women develop chronic insomnia. In addition, some perimenopausal and meno-pausal women deal with early-morning awakenings and intermittent sleep during the night. Fortunately, trouble falling asleep is the least common form of insomnia reported by women at this point in their lives. It is noteworthy, however, that complaints of insomnia are more common among women who do not use HRT. Insomnia is dis-cussed in detail in chapter 7.

Mood Changes

Perimenopausal women may have more anxiety and/or depressed feelings than they do at other times in their lives. Some-times these unsettling feelings preceding a hot flash can trigger an anxiety attack. For some women, disrupted or diminished sleep from hot flashes and other symptoms may contribute to their feeling more anxious and/or depressed during the day. At the same time, depressed, anxious, and/or stressed feelings, related or not to the perimenopausal years, may contribute to difficulty falling or remain-ing asleep during the night. Although anxiety usually resolves on its own without treatment, it may be a sign of a developing anxiety dis-order, such as panic disorder, which is distinguished by episodes of shortness of breath, chest pain, dizziness, heart palpitations, and/or feelings of "going crazy" or being out of control. Symptoms of anxi-ety can be related to depression as well. Treatments are available, so if you have significant, bothersome symptoms of anxiety, seek help for yourself. Relaxation and stress- reduction techniques, counseling, psychotherapy, and/or prescription drug treatment usually provide relief. (Depression, anxiety, etc., and sleep will be discussed at length in chapter 10.)

Respiratory Disturbance

After menopause, a woman's likelihood of developing sleep apnea increases. Sleep apnea is a serious condition in which breathing stops intermittently throughout the night. As a result, if you have sleep apnea, your sleep is disrupted and fragmented from repeated awakenings following the collapse of your airway. Not surprisingly, people with sleep apnea experience excessive daytime sleepiness.

The prevalence of sleep apnea, a form of sleep-disordered breathing (SDB), is estimated to be 9 percent for women and 24 percent for men between the ages of thirty and sixty. Sleep apnea becomes more common as both men and women age, with approximately 30 to 65 percent of elderly men and 20 to 55 percent of elderly women affected by SDB.

Following menopause, women are more likely to develop SDB (e.g., sleep apnea) than they are before they go through menopause (Guilleminault, Quera-Salva, Partinen, and Jamieson 1988). Moreover, sleep apnea in postmenopausal women tends to be more severe. This difference is probably due to falling progesterone levels in the older women, since younger women who experience surgical menopause (in which progesterone levels drop suddenly) are also at increased risk for developing sleep-disordered breathing. Higher body weight and lower levels of physical activity are also risk factors for this problem. The risk of SDB increases with age, although women are less susceptible at any age than men. Snoring, obesity, and high blood pressure are definite risk factors. Women may be under diagnosed for SDB because they may present with different symptoms than do men.

If you suspect that you or a family member may have sleep apnea, or even heavy snoring, I highly recommend that you be evaluated at a sleep disorders clinic. Studies have shown that even mild to moderate cases of SDB may be connected with serious health consequences, such as strokes, heart attacks, angina, and high blood pressure (Orr 1997). Chapter 8 includes an in-depth discussion of sleep apnea, its diagnosis, and its recommended treatment

Medial Treatment of Menopausal Symptoms

Changing levels of estrogen bring about many of the menopausal symptoms. Treatment with estrogen or a combination of estrogen and progesterone (hormone replacement therapy, or HRT) may relieve symptoms such as hot flashes and the significant sleep loss that results from them. However, women who take hormones such as HRT usually report more perimenopausal symptoms to begin with and, once treatment begins, they do not necessarily report fewer hot flashes or fewer awakenings (Lee and Taylor 1996). We also know that HRT decreases the risk of heart disease and osteoporosis (but taking HRT does not guarantee that you won't be affected by these diseases). Approximately 25 percent (8 million) of American menopausal women take HRT. The effects of HRT vary depending on the form taken (pill, patch, gel, cream, or injection) and the number of years used. One woman described what a profound difference HRT made in her life and in her sleep:

> My sleep was most disturbed during the menopause transition. This was due to the hot flashes that I was experiencing during the night. I would wake up in the middle of the night burning up and drenched in my own sweat. In the morning, I'd wake up and not feel at all refreshed. Although I was only thirty-nine, I realized that something was going on and got in touch with my gynecologist. After many tests, it was decided that I was indeed going through menopause and was put on hormone replacement therapy. Literally two days after going on medication, I felt like a new person. I have been on HRT close to four years now!

You (with your health-care provider) may want to consider using HRT for the following reasons: to reduce the symptoms of menopause, to reduce the risk of osteoporosis, and to reduce the risk of cardiovascular disease. The estrogen in HRT may help relieve many physical symptoms of menopause, such as hot flashes, vaginal dryness and irritation, urinary problems (e.g., muscle tone of the bladder, circulation to the urethra lining), unwanted hair growth, and problems with skin thickness and elasticity. In addition, sleep research has demonstrated that HRT can relieve symptoms such as hot flashes and therefore improve sleep efficiency, and decrease emotional instability (e.g., irritability and depressed mood), which sometimes accompany the physical symptoms of menopause (Greene, Lewis, Cabus, and Kletzky 1995; Moe 1999). Estrogen, because it reduces hot flashes, may allow a good night's rest, thereby decreasing irritability and other emotional difficulties.

Furthermore, it is evident that some waking episodes associated with menopause precede hot flashes by several minutes, and many waking episodes are not associated with hot flashes at all, but are related to SDB. Nonetheless, research has shown that ERT (estrogen alone) and HRT (estrogen plus progestin) may alleviate hot flashes as well as reduce apneic episodes in menopausal women diagnosed with sleep apnea, since HRT stimulates breathing during sleep (Keefe, Watson, and Naftolin 1999). However, taking progestin alone does not alleviate the sleep apnea (Block, Bush, White, Boysen, Wynne, and Taasan 1981).

However, HRT is not recommended for a number of women. Specifically, your health-care provider is not likely to recommend HRT if you have a personal or family history of breast cancer, blood clot in a vein (in the legs, lungs, or eyes), and/or liver disease. Perhaps the most serious risk associated with hormones, especially in long-term use, is the increased risk of cancer, particularly breast cancer (Colditz, Egan, and Stampfer 1993). Also, contrary to commonly held assumptions, the latest large-scale studies have found that women who already have coronary disease, such as blocked coronary arteries, are not protected from heart attacks or strokes by taking HRT (Simon, Hsia, Cauley, Richards, Harris, Fong, Barrett-Connor, and Hulley 2001). When considering HRT, women need to carefully review their own health history with their health-care practitioner. As you know, regardless of whether you take HRT, you'll face certain health risks and changes over the course of the perimenopausal and menopausal years.

Sleep-Smart Strategies during the Menopausal Transition

Here are some strategies that you may find helpful during the menopausal years. Regardless of whether you choose HRT as a way to deal with your menopausal symptoms, it is recommended that you consider multiple strategies.

* Eat healthfully. In general, it is beneficial for you to pay attention to your nutrition needs at this point (and indeed at every point) in your life. Specifically, increasing consumption of calcium and foods that promote absorption of calcium is a must during menopause, in order to protect against osteoporosis. Avoid eating very large meals, since they may trigger hot flashes. The following foods and other stimulants may also be triggers: spicy foods, acidic foods, caffeine, hot drinks, alcoholic drinks, saturated fats (e.g., meat and margarine), stress, hot weather, hot tubs and saunas, tobacco and marijuana, and overly intense exercise. Also, once a day eat at least one food rich in phytoestrogens, a weak form of estrogen found in soy products and some vegetables (e.g., squash, yams, and carrots). Soy foods, such as soy milk, soy yogurt, soy nuts, miso soup, tofu, and tempeh, seem to minimize or eliminate hot flashes.

* Exercise regularly. Exercise is a potent remedy for many meno-pausal complaints. Keep moving as much as possible. Regular physical activity and exercise relieve hot flashes, stress, and depressed mood, helping you in turn to sleep more efficiently. Furthermore, an exercise program that includes both aerobic and resistance training may prevent or lessen problems such as car-diovascular disease, obesity, osteoporosis, and depression. There are three types of exercise: aerobic, weight-bearing, and flexibil-ity. For greatest effect, do some of each of these kinds of exercises on a regular basis. Try to do at least thirty minutes of moderate aerobic exercise several days a week. Brisk walking for two miles is a good start. (I walk and/or jog two to four mornings a week with one or two close friends; this way I can exercise, catch up with friends, and get support at the same time.) Weight-bearing exercise (such as working out with weights) helps delay or pre-vent bone loss. Flexibility exercises are also important because they help you maintain function as you age. Check with your physician, nurse practitioner, or other health-care clinician to help you determine what level and type of exercise is appropriate for you at this time. Then find ways to fit exercise into your routine for the rest of your life. This is a commitment of time and energy that you deserve to make for yourself.

* Dress appropriately for sleep. Sleeping in a cool environment and in loose-fitting, lightweight clothes will improve your sleep effi-ciency in general and can significantly reduce the frequency and intensity of your hot flashes. Natural-fiber clothing may be more comfortable than synthetics; certainly, avoid sleeping in sweatpants or your new workout outfit.

* Reduce stress and worry. Of course, this is easier said than done! Some research suggests that hot flashes increase at times of stress. Fortunately, several studies have shown that women who prac-tice relaxation techniques experience a significant decrease in the intensity of their hot flashes, tension, and anxiety, as well as in their feelings of depressed mood (Domar and Dreher 1996). In particular, I recommend the progressive muscle relaxation (PMR) technique (Jacobson 1962), described in appendix B, in which you train yourself to gradually and systematically tense and relax groups of muscles. You can work this technique on your own or in consultation with a social worker, psychologist, or counselor. I recommend that you practice this technique approximately twenty minutes each day, for about six to eight weeks. After sev-eral weeks, you will notice that you are recovering more easily from your emotional stresses and strains and that your sleep effi-ciency is improved. During the first practice sessions each group

of muscles (forearm, upper arm, and so on) is exercised separately. Later these exercises are combined so that eventually you should be able to relax the whole body at once. It is likely that your first practice session will take about one hour (your daily training and the following sessions will take less than half this time). Women with acute or chronic pain (e.g., endometriosis, fibromyalgia, migraines, or severe back pain) may not wish to practice PMR, since it involves tensing of muscles and could bring on additional discomfort; instead, meditation, guided imagery, or listening to relaxation tapes or relaxing music may be more appropriate stress-reduction techniques. Finally, take time for yourself when you find that you are feeling stressed out, worried, irritated, or weepy. Get a massage; take a bath with a cup of herbal tea; laugh whenever you can. Establish a place where you can be alone, without responsibilities (well, without most responsibilities). For example, when my family and I moved recently, I insisted on having "a room of my own" in our new house. On the other hand, you may want to spend your sacred personal time with your close women friends. Generally take care of yourself when you're feeling stressed.

* Stick to a regular sleep routine. (Oh, yes, this book *is* about sleep!) Create a bedtime routine for yourself and try to go to bed close to the same time each night and get up around the same time each day.

* Consider using HRT. Talk with your health-care provider about HRT. Research definitely supports that estrogen supplements can make a significant difference in improving sleep for perimenopausal and menopausal women. (See Hormone Replacement Therapy, above, for more information.)

* Change your negative thinking. Try to label and replace distorted negative thoughts about menopause with positive, rational, truths. Specifically, ask yourself the following four questions: (1) Does this thought contribute to my stress? (2) Where did I learn this thought? (3) Is this thought logical? (4) Is this thought true? (Domar and Dreher 1996) Basically, break the negative menopause taboos. Talk with friends and family members about your hot flashes and other menopausal changes. Let people know when you are having a hot flash—this will reaffirm for you and others that there is nothing to be ashamed of. Use positive self-talk, even humor. Try attending a menopause support group or workshop as well.

* 6 *

Work, Motherhood, and Sleep

This chapter focuses on working women's sleep, or lack of sleep, a neglected health issue. This is a particularly relevant chapter for me because I am a working mother who often feels that I do not have enough time in the day to take a deep breath or enough time at night to sleep. This is a serious problem for me and for many women. Here is a typical day in my ridiculous schedule:

A Thursday in October

Rise time	5:37 A.M.
Fitness walk with close friend	5:50 to 6:40
Make coffee, get my son up, make his lunch (if not done the night before), drive or walk him part way to school	6:45 to 7:35
Get ready for work, get to my office	7:50 to 8:45
Teach my first class Grade papers, return calls, e-mail	9:30 to 10:45
Prepare for next class, grab a snack/lunch	11:00 A.M. to 12:30 P.M.
Teach second class	12:30 to 1:45
Hold student office hours Try to get some writing done	2:00 to 3:30
Return phone calls for volunteer work	3:45 to 5:00
Pick up my son at afterschool program	by 5:15

Take him to his hockey practice; then head home with him to join my husband (usually he has made dinner!)	5:30 to 7:00
(Hope I don't have an evening meeting), eat dinner	7:15 to 8:00
Help my son with homework	8:00 to 8:30
Go through bedtime routines, put my son to bed	8:45 to 9:00
Make phone calls for my volunteer activities, and personal calls, grade papers, crash time—television, read the paper	9:00 to 10:00
Exhaustion, sleep!	10:30 (if I'm lucky)

Here is how, a longtime friend of mine poignantly portrayed her experience with sleep as a woman with a career, marriage, and children:

I am so tired that when my head hits the pillow, I take a deep breath, and that is the last thing I remember. With a start, I awaken, panicked, by a slamming door. It is my teenage son, arriving home. All is well. I pat my chest to calm my rapid heartbeat. Okay. All is well. I can sleep now. It takes a few minutes to recover from the jolt, but I am so exhausted that sleep comes again.

What? Is this a dream? No, my husband has gotten up in the middle of the night. What time is it? No, it is not time to get up yet. All is well. I try to go back to sleep, but this time it is harder. My mind is beginning to focus on the events of the day to come. I breathe deeply in an effort to calm my racing mind. I know I need my sleep. I cannot get comfortable. I try so hard to go back to sleep.

Next, there is a knock at the door. Did I even fall back asleep? "Mommy, I had a nightmare." I wonder if this is all a conspiracy. After getting my young daughter back to bed at three o'clock, I contemplate just staying up. But I need my sleep, I must try to sleep some more. It is hard, though. I am agitated, angry, anxious, and still exhausted.

As I stated in the introduction to this book, the Women's Bureau of the U.S. Department of Labor reported, in its survey of over a quarter of a million women, that the majority of working women say that stress and fatigue are their primary struggles. So it is not surprising that working women report increased fatigue and greater use of sleeping pills than men do (Jacquinet-Salord, Lang, Fouriaud, Nicoulet, and Bingham 1993). Other researchers found that full-time employed mothers of young children tend to forgo personal care, good sleep habits, and leisure time (Walker and Best 1991). Other studies have shown that women who have more rewarding relationships with partners and/or children report lower levels of fatigue and other health problems. There remain numerous unanswered questions regarding fatigue, sleepiness levels, and sleep schedules of working women.

In this chapter, I review some of the issues that have been investigated by psychologists and other researchers regarding the intricate relationship between work, motherhood, health, sleep, and mental health. Later in the chapter, I share some findings from a survey study of working women's sleep-wake patterns that I conducted a few years ago. Finally, at the conclusion of the chapter, I again present Sleep-Smart Strategies.

Women in the Workplace

According to the U.S. Department of Labor, Women's Bureau (1999), over 60 percent of women work, and over 75 percent of them work full-time (thirty-five hours per week or more). Women ages thirty-five to forty-four had the highest labor participation rates compared to other age groups in 1999, and women, as single parents, maintained 13 million of the 71 million families in the United States in 1998.

Employment and Women's Health

Research indicates that employment is associated with both health advantages and disadvantages. Researchers reviewed close to forty studies of the effects of employment on women's psychological well-being, and they found either positive effects or no differences associated with employment (Warr and Parry 1982). Other psychologists have reported that employment is actually associated with lower rates of depression in women. Similarly, women with multiple roles, such as employee and mother, reported that they were healthier than women with fewer roles did (Verbrugge 1983). These studies emphasize that having multiple roles may buffer women against depression, low self-esteem, perceptions of poor health, and other psychosocial health factors.

On the other hand, researchers have reported that employment detracts from healthy lifestyles. For example, in one study employed mothers reported more perceived stress and less healthy lifestyles than nonemployed mothers did (Walker and Best 1991). The main sources of stress for nonemployed women were fatigue, sleep disturbances, and work overload. Full-time employed mothers reported conflicts about going back to work, lack of time, fatigue, and sleep disturbances.

Not surprisingly, employed mothers reported that they had less time to relax, to eat three regular meals a day, and to engage in physical exercise than did nonemployed mothers. Nonetheless, nearly 50 percent of nonemployed mothers (versus over 70 percent of employed mothers) reported that they rarely took some time in their day for these self-care activities. The results of this study indicate that non-employed mothers are only somewhat more likely to attend to their own personal health and well-being than nonemployed mothers are.

One well-known study concluded that working women are dual-shift workers. The study found that after putting in eight hours or more at work, women return home to complete a second shift—family responsibilities. This second shift has negative effects on women's health (Hochschild 1989). In the Working Women Count survey (U. S. Department of Labor, Women's Bureau 1994), women clearly emphasized that it is very difficult to balance work demands and family responsibilities in today's workplace-driven culture. Working mothers' total sleep times and sleep- wake schedules may be very different from those of men or women without children in the home because of this double workday, or because of single parenthood.

Work and Sleep-Wake Patterns

Fatigue, exhaustion, and sleep disturbances are common problems for many working women. For example in a sample of just over four hundred working women, 86 percent of the women complained of fatigue and exhaustion (Barnett, Davidson, and Marshall 1991). Women surveyed by the Women's Bureau of the U.S. Department of Labor (1994) for the *Report to the Nation* ranked stress and fatigue as their number one problem. This problem was identified by 60 percent of the women from a range of income and occupational groups. It was particularly acute for women in their forties who hold professional and managerial jobs (74 percent). Clearly, working women consider fatigue and sleep disturbances to be among their primary sources of stress.

Studies on women's sleep are providing an emerging picture of the sleep-related issues that are particularly important to working women. Fatigue, often a symptom of disturbed sleep, is more prevalent among women than men (Alward and Monk 1990; Barnett, Davidson, and Marshall 1991). In the sample of more than four hundred working women mentioned above, 86 percent complained of fatigue and exhaustion and 64 percent noted that they had trouble sleeping (Barnett, Davidson, and Marshall 1991). Women, particularly those over age forty-five, complain of more sleep problems than do men (Lugaresi, Mondini, Zucconi, Montagna, and Cirignotta 1983); and consumption of sleeping tablets is particularly high among women (11 percent among women, 6 percent among men (Jacquinet-Salord, Lang, Fouriaud, Nicoulet, and Bingham 1993). Sleeping-tablet consumption and sleep-disturbance reports were higher among participants who said they had a negative work atmosphere and increased time pressures.

One of my close friends reflected on how exhausted she felt while working full-time with two children under the age of three:

> I returned to work three months after having each of my children. I was older than most women are when they have children—I had just turned forty—and I feel this has something to do with the fact that I was so tired all of the time. I could literally feel and see myself aging after the second child. I remember driving to work and crying because I was so worn out. I wondered if I had cancer or some other serious disease. My speech was also disrupted at this point in my life—I can remember calling objects by the wrong name. When this would happen at work and in meetings, I would feel quite embarrassed. My most salient issue of being a mother was my complete exhaustion. I recall not being able to pick up my feet and just shuffling around the house on weekends. I felt as if something was wrong with me. I could not take the fatigue any longer. Some of my friends recommended taking vitamins, which I did, and it helped me to feel better. I know that being a working mother had a lot to do with my tiredness because I was not at liberty to take a nap during the day. Even on the weekends, I could not nap because I had a toddler and a baby to care for. My husband was exhausted also, but we both felt we should be there for each other, and we did not nap because of that.

Working mothers with school-age children are increasingly more likely to choose night-shift work as opposed to working day or evening shifts in order to be compensated at a higher rate, to lower child-care costs, and to maximize time with their partners and children (Garey 1999). Dr. Kathy Lee and others have focused their research on shift workers, such as nurses, and women with particular sleep disturbances. Lee (1992) examined female nurses working night, evening, and rotating shifts. She found that there were more sleep problems and difficulties staying awake during shifts in nurses working permanent nights and rotating shifts, and that permanent night nurses thought that they got less sleep than did the nurses on the other shifts. All of the women reported more sleep on their days off than during workdays (Lee 1992). Sociologist Anita Garey interviewed several nurses in her 1999 book, *Weaving Work and Motherhood*. The nurses working the night shift reported experiencing serious sleep deprivation and a range of compromises in their lives. For example, one woman reported skipping an entire day of sleep so she could make her daughter's costume for an upcoming dance recital. Never-ending lack of sleep and continually feeling exhausted while spending time with one's family often forces women to seek other schedules, if they are fortunate to get such opportunities, or to leave their night-shift jobs all together.

Sleep and Daytime Functioning

If you are a sleepy or fatigued woman, you are probably more likely than women who are not fatigued to encounter difficulties during the day or report irritability or other mood fluctuations. In our fast-paced culture, we seem to expect individuals to somehow make their sleep accommodate their work and family schedules. With regular sleep, most people are alert, cheerful, and active; their sleepiness, like wakefulness, is normal and cyclic. Too little sleep disturbs the normal sleep-wake cycle and may lead to impaired performance when working (Webb 1992). Problems due to irregular schedules and inadequate sleep—fatigue at work, diminished cognitive abilities, industrial accidents, depressed mood, irritability, lethargy, and related sleep disturbances—have been documented by numerous sleep researchers. For example, college men and women with irregular sleep schedules who made regular their sleep schedules but experienced sleep loss in the process reported an increase in daytime sleepiness and a simultaneous deterioration in mood and concentration (Manber and Bootzin 1991). Similarly, medical residents reported associations between sleep loss, erratic sleep-wake schedules, negative self-perception, and depressed mood (Tanz and Charrow 1993). Furthermore, inattentiveness from sleep deprivation may result in serious injuries at work or while driving a car, as well as less dramatic problems such as struggling to remain alert while helping your child with homework. Although fatigue is a major complaint voiced by working women, it is not evident what is meant by fatigue, and how it is associated with daytime functioning. In one of my studies, we assessed the relationship between working women's sleep-wake patterns and their reports of depressed mood and overall malaise.

A Survey of Working Women's Sleep

In fall 1995, I administered the Women's Sleep and Health Questionnaire to women working daytime shifts at corporations, businesses, and schools in Massachusetts and Rhode Island. Participants completed the survey at their job sites. The survey items queried working women about usual sleeping and waking behaviors over the previous two weeks (see appendix B).

The survey was completed anonymously by nearly two hundred women. Women's ages ranged from twenty-two to fifty-eight years. Sixty-eight percent of the sample were married, and 32 percent were separated, divorced, or single. Ninety-two percent of the women were Caucasian and 8 percent were of other races. Fifty- five percent of the sample had children aged eighteen or under living at home. Of the mothers in the group, the largest number had small children.

The women surveyed in the Women's Sleep and Health Questionnaire were working long hours. Seventy percent reported that they worked 35 hours or more each week. In addition, 35 percent brought five to twenty hours of office work home per week. Fifty percent reported that they spent twenty hours or more per week on household/family responsibilities. The majority of these women noted that they usually left home at 7:30 A.M. or earlier to get to work, and 34 percent worked until 5:30 P.M. or later.

Nearly 80 percent of the women surveyed reported that they needed 8 or more hours of sleep each night in order to feel their best every day. However, many of them were not getting those eight hours every night. Thirty-two percent of the women reported that they slept less than 6.5 hours on weeknights (average of 7 hours, 3 minutes), and nearly 30 percent slept less than 7.5 hours on weekend nights (average of 8 hours, 6 minutes). Just over 60 percent of the women reported that their weeknight bedtimes were between 10:00 and 11:00 P.M., and 85 percent of them said they woke up at 6:30 A.M. or earlier. The women noted that they went to bed on weekends an average of about 50 minutes later and started their days nearly 2 hours later. Most of the women reported that it took them less than 20 minutes, on average, to fall asleep each night. During the week, these women did not have much time for naps; however, 40 percent reported that they take weekend naps.

For the women surveyed, the amount of sleep they got was significantly affected by their number of work hours. Specifically, women working 35 hours or more per week reported 20 minutes less sleep each night than women working fewer hours. In fact, just over 40 percent of the full-time employed women reported that they got less than 6.5 hours of sleep per night during the week. However, full-time employed women had relatively consistent weekend-weekday bedtime schedules, whereas part-timers went to bed more than an hour later on weekends. This finding that so many women working full-time are sleeping less than 6.5 hours per night during the workweek helps to explain why fatigue is reported as working women's primary concern (Women's Bureau of the U.S. Department of Labor 1994, *Working Women Count Survey*). The bottom line is that we do not have enough time to sleep.

So, what are the consequences? Regardless of age, parental status, and number of work hours, women who reported having less time for sleep acknowledged increased levels of depressed mood and overall malaise in comparison to longer sleepers. Likewise, working women with more irregular sleep schedules (e.g., greater differences between weeknight and weekend bedtimes) experienced depressed mood and malaise. These data strongly suggest that working women with inadequate total sleep and/or irregular sleep schedules experience more moodiness and emotional distress.

Are there certain kinds of responsibilities or tasks that may be more affected by sleep loss? Although sleep researchers have not examined this specific question, researchers Rosalind Barnett and Carol Rivers (1996) examined the impact of different types of tasks on other aspects of men's and women's lives. They found that men and women are working very long hours, at least 70 hours a week doing paid work and household chores. Similarly, our sample reported that they spent an average of 72 hours a week on paid office work, take-home work, and household responsibilities. In Barnett and Rivers's study, mental health was studied in connection with the type of tasks being done as opposed to how long the tasks took. The researchers described low-control tasks as those tasks for which one has little control over when they must be done, such as feeding the family and buying groceries, and high control tasks as those that do not have to be done at a specific time, such as making house repairs, doing yard work, and taking out the garbage. They found that at home women spent more time on low-control tasks, whereas men did more of the high-control tasks; low-control tasks were associated with greater distress than high-control ones. In addition, they noted that full-time employed women in the sample reported less stress than both the unemployed and part-time employed women did because full-time working women engaged in more high-control activities (at their job sites) (Barnett and Rivers 1996). Barnett and Rivers's findings suggest that stress is associated more with certain types of tasks than with the number of hours worked. Our survey study indicates that increased work hours are associated with less total sleep. From these findings, it may be hypothesized that distress from insufficient sleep may interfere more with jobs that must be done everyday as opposed to tasks that may be put on hold for a while.

Researchers and clinicians are beginning to understand the complex association between emotional well-being and sleep patterns. (See chapter 10 for a close look at the relationship between mental health and sleep-wake patterns in women.) Because of this association between sleep and emotional health, it is important that working women practice intervention and prevention strategies that help to improve their sleep.

Conclusions

The implications of these data seem undeniable. First, women—you and I—need to take an active role and examine our sleep habits as they relate to work and family responsibilities, mood fluctuations, personal time, and self-care. Second, investigators and practitioners in other health-care fields need to pay closer attention to sleep as a factor in women's health.

It is clear that full-time working women require more than 6.8 hours (sample mean) of sleep to cope with work demands, family responsibilities, driving, and other stressors. Although different women may be differently affected by work and family responsibilities, insufficient, erratic sleep is a potentially serious factor in women's health care and emotional well-being. The extent of the problem has gone unrecognized because sleepiness is so prevalent that it almost seems normal (Carskadon 1990; Mitler, Dement, and Dinges 2000).

Sleep-Smart Strategies for Working Women

To help you combat sleep problems in your own life, below are some specific Sleep-Smart Strategies for working women who have a range of additional responsibilities, such as caring for children or aging parents.

* Balance your life. Set priorities. Identify a specific personal bedtime and stick to it. In other words, try to go to bed and wake up at the same time every day. I realize that this is easier said than done, especially for working mothers, but do try to identify some ways you could clear your evening and early-morning schedule—cut back on those evening calls to friends and family members, avoid checking your e-mail at night, or turn off the television earlier, for example. Establishing a regular pattern will

set your internal body clock. Schedule a nightly transition time so that you can relax (e.g., take a bath, read, or listen to music before going to bed). Avoid strenuous or stressful activities before bed, such as planning for the next day, paying bills, or exercising.

* Use caffeine wisely. Although women and men have consumed caffeinated foods and beverages for hundreds of years, questions persist about its potential effects on women's health. According to leading medical and scientific experts, caffeine consumed in moderation produces no adverse health effects. However, caffeine is a mild stimulant that affects many areas in the body, including the brain. In sufficient quantity—one hundred milligrams or one cup of coffee—caffeine increases neural activity in many parts of the brain. It increases performance of simple intellectual tasks, enhances rapid processing of information, causes increased alertness and ability to concentrate. Caffeine also increases endurance and counters sleepiness, and it usually delays the onset of sleep. Studies have also shown that it reduces the length, depth, and quality of sleep. Users exhibit more movement during sleep and are more easily awoken. So, as I've discussed earlier in the book it's best to avoid caffeine within four to six hours of bedtime.

* Help your body adjust to night-shift or on-call work. Women night-shift workers report that they get less sleep and that their sleep is more disrupted than that of their brothers, spouses, and fathers on similar work schedules. If you are married and you both work the night shift, you probably have less time available to sleep than your husband does. If you work a late- or night-shift or on-call schedule, you probably find yourself trying to sleep when your body wants to be awake and having to be awake when your body wants to sleep. Workers who are most affected are those who work nights and those on rotating shift patterns. There is evidence that these workers are at risk for more sleep-related accidents and illnesses, such as colds. In addition, you may find that your family life is strained due to conflicting sleep times, lack of sleep, or feeling like you cannot contribute to family activities. Night-shift work may also add to your stress by making it difficult to pursue ordinary leisure activities, help your children with homework, meet friends, make medical appointments, and do chores and errands.

    Your goal should be to sleep as well as is possible when off duty and be alert when working. Rotating shifts should when possible be rotated clockwise so that you go from day shift to evening shift to night shift. This minimizes sleep deprivation as well as circadian clock disruption. Research has shown that shift patterns that are planned with circadian factors in mind tend to help workers be more productive, feel happier, and have fewer accidents. Rest periods during shifts may increase alertness, possibly decreasing tiredness and enhancing productivity. Talk with your employer to optimize scheduling.

Do your best to adopt a fixed sleep time, going to bed and getting up at about the same time no matter when you're working. Clearly this is impossible for those working intermittent night shifts. However, if you're on a permanent night-shift schedule, you will feel and perform better if you sleep by day even during nights off. If you're on an early or late shift, without any overnight work, you should try to go to sleep at the same time each night. If you're on a rotating shift, you may cope better if you plan your sleep times carefully as a scheduling change approaches. For example, for a few nights before moving from a late to a night shift, delay your bedtimes and rise times for one or two hours each night. You will then be well on your way adapting to the new schedule when you begin a long-term night shift schedule. Also, if you are scheduled on an on-call rotation (for example, if you are a physician or nurse), try to stay ahead of the game with a regular sleep-wake schedule so that you go into the on-call period as rested as possible. Finally, naps can be refreshing and should be taken when you feel excessively sleepy. However, those experiencing difficulties with sleeping when in bed should be careful not to nap so much that they reduce the body's drive to sleep when they get to bed.

*   Protect your nighttime and naptime sleep. Historically, nappers (particularly women) have been labeled by society as lazy and unmotivated. This has to change. Working women and working mothers need sleep just as much as other people. Say "yes" to sleep even when you're tempted to stay up late or skip your afternoon nap (e.g., to watch a favorite old movie on television, to talk to an old friend, to fold laundry, to work, or to watch the kids so your partner can nap). Try to deal with worries and distractions several hours before going to bed. In addition, silence or quiet sounds are essential for quality sleep. Fall asleep to music only if it is nondistracting and uninterrupted by radio announcers—who can scare you out of an otherwise good sleep! Some women may find the low humming of a fan, humidifier, or air conditioner to be helpful. Heavy curtains can muffle outside noise, and your telephone, pager, and computer can always be turned off!

*   Share sleep with your partner. In other words, do not skimp on sleep just so that your partner can get his or her sleep. Many women whom I have interviewed over the years have commented on how their spouses seem to have no difficulty napping in a

variety of places (e.g., in front of the television or at their desks) and at various times of day (e.g., weekend afternoons or early weekday evenings). These women have told me that they are often busy organizing for the next day, helping with homework, putting children to bed, and doing other tasks while their spouse naps! It is crucial that you and your partner make sleep a priority for both of you. Talk to your partner and ask for his support; together, work out a sleep schedule that allows for weekend naps, taking turns getting the children ready for school, and even sharing in the children's bedtime rituals, so that one or both of you can get to bed earlier.

Make sure your sleep conditions, including your bed, are as comfortable as possible. If you share your bed with a snoring, cover-stealing, or restless partner, you may want to make temporary separate sleeping arrangements until you establish a satisfactory sleeping pattern.

* Exercise regularly, but not instead of sleeping. A good exercise program during the day, at least four hours before bedtime, can be helpful for a good night's sleep. However, exercise is not a substitute for sleep. A number of my friends love to walk early in the morning, before their children get up for school. Keeping this sort of regular exercise schedule is admirable; however, sometimes exercising so early in the morning instead of sleeping may be doing more (in a negative direction) for your sleep debt than benefitting your cardiovascular system.

* Learn techniques for coping with sleep deprivation. There are a variety of behavioral and practical strategies that are helpful when you are sleep deprived. First, taking naps is a great way to recharge your batteries. Try taking a fifteen-minute nap break, even at work. Second, if you have been skimping on sleep and cannot reschedule several projects, meetings, or other commitments, tackle your most challenging task when you are most alert (you may feel most alert in the morning, whereas other women have the most energy in the afternoon and evening). Similarly, save your least demanding projects for the time you're most likely to be tired. Also, try to avoid getting into situations that are emotionally draining. Don't let minor hassles turn into full-blown confrontations. Take a couple of deep breaths and think before you speak. Finally, simplify your daily routine. For example, my husband and I both do the laundry, but when we are tired and busy, we do not put the clothes away. Instead, we stack them in separate piles on shelves near the washing machine and each of us (including our nine-year-old son) manages to find what we are looking for each day.

✳ Think positively about napping (unless you struggle with insomnia). I highly recommend reading *The Art of Napping at Work* by Camille and Bill Anthony (1999). In their book, they outline the following habits for effective workplace napping:

(a) Plan and announce your naps to yourself and to your colleagues, if possible. This step will reinforce positive feelings about the napping concept.

(b) Gather napping tools or items that will help promote napping (for example, you may want to store a favorite blanket or pillow in your desk or closet).

(c) Keep your nap regular and timed. In other words, it is helpful to try to nap at approximately the same time and for the same total amount of time each day. Therefore, you may need to bring an alarm clock to your office or even take turns with a close colleague to wake each other up.

(d) Ensure control of your nap environment so that you are not interrupted and awakened prematurely. You may want to shut off the phone, have your calls held, find a secret nap spot, close your door (if possible) and put up a sign that says, "Break in progress," "Nap time," "No interruptions please," or "Will return in x minutes."

(e) Prevent sleep inertia. Sleep inertia is that groggy, disoriented feeling that some people may experience when they awaken. Research suggests that if you nap for forty to sixty minutes you are more likely to awaken from deep sleep and therefore experience this sleep inertia. However, if you take a twenty- to thirty-minute power nap or a ninety- to one hundred-minute (long-duration) nap you will be less likely to experience this grogginess.

(f) Celebrate your napping habit.

✳ Consider using light therapy. Human beings are influenced by light. Light determines our sleep-wake cycle. Your rhythm of being alternately asleep and awake can be reversed or advanced by means of light exposure. For instance, a worker who gets thirty minutes to one hour of bright-light therapy before a night shift can postpone her heavy fatigue, normally occurring between two and five o'clock in the morning, until dawn. Correspondingly, bright-light therapy in the morning reduces daytime fatigue.

✳ Educate your employer and colleagues about the importance of sleep. As you now know, an optimal shift schedule promotes higher company morale, lower job turnover, higher productivity, fewer errors, and lower absenteeism (Monk and Wagner 1989; Moore-Ede 1998). Researchers have documented the steps that employers can take to help their workers cope with shift work, particularly so that they are not sleep deprived (Moore-Ede 1998; Smolensky and Lamberg 2000; National Institute for Occupational Safety and Health 1997). If you are employed by a company or institution that relies on shifts or long work hours, I highly recommend that you begin to dialogue with your employer and colleagues about making the following changes:

* adopting schedules that rotate clockwise (i.e., from morning to night), thereby preventing abrupt shift changes for employees;

* educating employees regarding sleep, diet, exercise, and drug use (including cigarettes and alcohol);

* providing some sort of twenty-four-hour access to a store or restaurant that serves healthy snacks and meals;

* installing exercise equipment so that you and your colleagues can exercise during breaks regardless of work schedule;

* providing frequent breaks and arrange comfortable areas for on-site napping;

* developing cross-training and job-sharing so that you and your coworkers can do a variety of tasks and have more job flexibility;

* providing health awareness programs for new workers and their families;

* and offering on-site child care for extended weekday and weekend hours (for example, one daycare company, Children's Choice, has set up six employer-sponsored round-the-clock child-care programs in the United States and will open more in the next three years).

* 7 *

Sleep Problems for
Women: Insomnia

Nearly everyone experiences poor or insufficient sleep at one time or another. Poor sleep or lack of sleep often comes at a time when you've experienced some sort of change in your life, leaving you feeling tired, fatigued, foggy, and/or unable to keep your eyes open during the day. Luckily, for most people, this change in their sleep-wake pattern is temporary and should cause minimal concern. However, for some people, sleep struggles are chronic, more severe, and may warrant attention from a health-care provider. In this chapter, I focus on the complaint of insomnia, the most common sleep symptom encountered by the general population, especially women.

In the National Sleep Foundation's Women and Sleep Poll (1998), 53 percent of the women surveyed reported having had one or more insomnia symptoms in the past month, 35 percent noted that they felt unrefreshed upon awakening, over 30 percent of the women reported that they had used over-the-counter and/or prescription sleep aids during the past year, and 8 percent made use of alcohol for the same purpose. Twenty to 50 percent of the women reported having difficulty concentrating or feeling foggy during the day.

The medical, scientific, and lay communities have discussed insomnia, often considered the common cold of sleep disorders, for at least two thousand years, beginning with Aristotle's monograph on sleeplessness, written in 350 B.C.E. Research indicates that up to 40 percent of adults report at least occasional difficulty sleeping. Chronic insomnia affects nearly 10 to 15 percent of the adult population (National Sleep Foundation 2000, *Treating Insomnia in the Primary Care Setting*). Insomnia occurs in men and women of all age groups, although it seems to be more common in women (especially after menopause) and in the elderly. Specifically, 1.5 to 2 times more women report insomnia than do men. In general, the ability to sleep, rather than the need for sleep, appears to decrease with advancing age. Research suggests that approximately 30 percent of adults over age sixty-five struggle with insomnia.

Insomnia is the most commonly reported sleep problem, not only in the United States, but also in industrialized countries around the world (Chesson, Hartse, Anderson, Davila, Johnson, Littner, Wise, and Rafecas 2000). Although insomnia seems to affect large numbers of people (particularly women), most do not seek professional advice or treatment. Unfortunately, however, chronic insomnia may be associated with a perceived decrease in quality of life, an increase in physical complaints, economic consequences including decreased work productivity, and an increase in car and occupational accidents (Sateia, Doghramji, Hauri, and Morin 2000). In addition, research suggests that there are medical risks associated with decreased sleep time and with chronic use of sleeping pills (Kripke, Klauber, Wingard, Fell, Assmus, and Garfinkel 1998).

What Is Insomnia, Anyway?

Although insomnia seems to be a very common problem, it continues to be under diagnosed and poorly understood by sufferers and clinicians alike. Defining insomnia is not a simple task. The word *insomnia* comes from Latin and its direct translation is "no sleep." Yet, when we discuss insomnia we usually mean difficulty sleeping, not enough sleep, and/or sleep with poor quality. Researchers and clinicians define insomnia as inadequate or poor-quality sleep due to one or more of the following: difficulty falling asleep, waking up frequently during the night with difficulty returning to sleep, waking up too early in the morning, and/or unrefreshing sleep. Insomnia may cause problems during the day, such as tiredness, lack of energy, difficulty concentrating, and irritability. Neither the number of hours of sleep a person gets nor the amount of time it takes to fall asleep indicates insomnia. Individuals vary normally in their need for, and their satisfaction with, sleep.

Insomnia can be classified as *transient* (short-term), *intermittent*, and *chronic*. Insomnia lasting from a single night to a few weeks is referred to as transient. If episodes of transient insomnia occur from time to time, the insomnia is said to be intermittent. Insomnia is considered to be chronic if it occurs on three or more nights per week and lasts three months or more. It is crucial to understand that insomnia is not a disease—it is really a symptom, like a fever or joint pain, that requires a careful examination. A sleep- laboratory assessment may, or may not, verify your sense that your sleep is being curtailed.

Each individual may experience somewhat different symptoms and/or types of insomnia. In fact, your primary symptoms may vary widely in type, intensity, frequency, the factors that cause them, and daytime consequences. The most obvious way to categorize insomnia is by the time of night when sleep problems are most bothersome. One common type of insomnia is sleep-onset insomnia, or trouble falling asleep at the beginning of the night (Lacks 1987)—you may have trouble falling asleep, yet once you do fall asleep the remainder of your night is not necessarily disrupted. A second type of disturbed sleep is sleep-maintenance insomnia, or sleep that is interrupted in the middle of the night—you may awaken in the middle of the night (perhaps more than once) and have difficulty falling back to sleep. A third type is early-morning awakening, when you wake up before your desired rise time. In addition to suffering from one of these types of insomnia, you may also experience sleep that seems light, restless, disturbed, and/or unreliable throughout the week or month. Insomnia-like difficulties may also be categorized according to intensity. In the sections below, I define these variations of insomnia.

Transient Insomnia

Everyone experiences this sort of insomnia, by definition, from time to time. This sort of sleep difficulty lasts for a few nights, about a week at most. It is often associated with a specific event. For example, I vividly recall experiencing difficulty falling asleep and staying asleep during the first few nights after my mother died a few years ago. The experience was very stressful, but the insomnia slowly went away. Perhaps you have had difficulty sleeping the night before an important exam when you were in college. Transient insomnia is also common after a time-zone change and is one of the symptoms of jet lag. However, you certainly do not have to travel far to experience insomnia. You may find that you have transient insomnia when you sleep in a different or unfamiliar place for the first few nights of a holiday. With transient insomnia, however, normal sleep usually returns within a few days. The treatment for transient insomnia depends on the circumstances. For the most part, no intervention is necessary other than remembering that having difficulty sleeping can be normal, and trying not to worry about it.

Short-Term Insomnia

Some people experience insomnia for a few weeks. If this is the case for you, then you probably have short-term insomnia. Similar to transient insomnia, short-term insomnia symptoms often start after a stressful life event, such as a divorce, the death of a loved one, or the loss of a job. In all likelihood, you may find that as you resolve the emotional issues surrounding the life event, your sleep improves as well. However, people may develop poor sleep habits and anxiety about sleep at this time. Sometimes, this leads to more chronic forms of insomnia. Note that if you experience what you think is short-term insomnia but have not had any obvious worries or stressful life event to account for it, you may have another sleep disorder, such as sleep apnea or periodic leg movements in sleep (see chapter 8).

Chronic Insomnia

If your insomnia lasts for a minimum of three months, then you are probably experiencing chronic insomnia. Insomnia sometimes lasts for years, graduating from transient to short-term to chronic. Perhaps you have resolved the issues or gotten past the event(s) that caused your initial insomnia complaints, but the insomnia remains. Many clinicians refer to this as *conditioned* or *psychophysiological insomnia*. Chronic insomnia is not always prompted by a stressful event. Specifically, insomnia symptoms may begin with a physical illness, depression, or anxiety. They may stem from poor sleep habits, such as the use or abuse of caffeine, alcohol, and/or sleeping pills, or from trying to sleep in a non-sleep-promoting environment (e.g., where there is too much noise or light).

There is no absolute definition of insomnia that is accepted by all clinicians (e.g., psychologists and physicians), sleep researchers, and other health-care professionals. However, the following description for primary insomnia (insomnia that is not the result of another health problem) is:

* Difficulty initiating or maintaining sleep for a minimum of three months (sleep latency of thirty minutes or more for three or more nights per week)

* Sleep efficiency (i.e., amount of time asleep relative to total time in bed) less than or equal to 85 percent

* Sleep disturbance associated with experience of daytime fatigue accompanied by mood and performance difficulties at home or work

* Sleep disturbance not due to other sleep disorder, such as narcolepsy, apnea, or circadian rhythm disorder

* Sleep disturbance does not occur exclusively during mental health problem, such as depression, or anxiety disorder

* Sleep disturbance not due to effects of alcohol, medication, or other medical condition

What Causes and Maintains Insomnia?

Disentangling the chain of factors that may contribute to your insomnia symptoms entails looking at the pre-insomnia picture of your sleep, the initial symptoms, any changes over time, and your current sleep-wake patterns. Causes of insomnia may be physical or psychological, or some combination of the two. While sometimes related to a physical disorder or advancing age, insomnia is more often than not related to emotional distress, since thoughts of self-reproach often become magnified in the late evening and early morning hours. Some common physical causes of insomnia include the normal physiological changes experienced in aging; respiratory abnormalities (such as sleep apnea, in which airways become temporarily blocked); leg cramps; ulcer-related pain; the need to urinate; and discomforts of pregnancy.

Other common cases include stressful life events, depression, anxiety, jet lag, alcohol, and certain drugs and food. Here is how a close friend of mine described her experience with insomnia:

> About two and a half years ago, I had an amazing spell of insomnia after flying to Europe. Even though everyone who flew with me was experiencing a period of jet lag and time adjustment, mine was much more severe. I do not remember sleeping at all the first day. I felt as if I had not slept for nine days in a row. I felt like I was walking around in a haze, like a zombie. When I returned from my trip overseas, I slept better, but some problems persisted. For a few months, I had trouble staying asleep. I would wake up all night long. Books about insomnia instructed me not to lie awake for more than fifteen minutes. Therefore, I would read something boring when I felt I had been lying awake too long. I would always be reading at about one in the morning. For a few weeks, this tactic helped my sleep to improve. I asked my doctor about taking medication for insomnia. However, he discouraged me from taking sleeping pills and instructed me to take Benadryl [antihistamine] to help me to fall asleep. The Benadryl did not help my sleep at all. I just sat in bed feeling spacey and odd, and in the morning I felt very groggy.
>
> My job as a nurse has certainly contributed to my sleep problems. When I anticipate having a bad day, I usually have

trouble sleeping the night before. For example, one time when things were really crazy at work, I knew I was going to have an awful day the next day. I knew I would really need to be alert. I was exhausted, but I was unable to sleep well, partly because I knew I needed to sleep, and partly due to stress. As it turned out, the next day was hard, but my functioning was fine. I never have headaches due to lack of sleep. Also, since my job is very physical, I rarely get sleepy on the job, and my daily functioning is rarely impaired. However, when I get home, the adrenaline wears off. I usually take a nap at around four or five o'clock in the afternoon, even though my husband often suggests that I will not fall asleep at night if I nap. I have a habit of going to bed around nine or ten o'clock at night, and I never watch television before I go to bed, but I often read. I now have the conditioned response to initially feel sleepy when I read a book, but after a few minutes of reading I feel wide awake and can't easily get to sleep.

Even though sleep has not been one of my greatest gifts, I do okay with the sleep I get, and I am not suffering too much. I have now lost the fear of not being able to fall asleep because I have realized that I can still continue to survive and function with the small amount of sleep I do get.

Current research demonstrates that insomnia is often a chronic condition that goes undiagnosed and untreated. Surveys indicate that approximately 80 percent of those with more severe insomnia have suffered from their symptoms for more than one year, and about 40 percent of insomnia sufferers report that they have had the condition for more than five years. In the paragraphs below, I describe the predisposing factors (those that make a person more susceptible), precipitating factors (variables that trigger initial symptoms), and perpetuating factors (behaviors and situations that cause the problem to continue) that contribute to the development of insomnia. Many of these descriptions will be familiar to you and may help you begin to make changes in your life that will lead to reducing, mitigating, or treating your insomnia.

Predisposing Factors

Psychologists define predisposing factors as conditions that set the stage for insomnia and influence whether the problem will become more chronic (Spielman and Glovinsky 1997). Individuals who tend to worry a lot and are anxious and emotional may be more inclined to develop insomnia-like symptoms. Night owls, people who have lots of energy at night and dread the morning, also seem to be more likely to have sleep-onset difficulties; night-owl behavior may contribute to the development of insomnia. For example, a friend of mine takes a nap from about half past eight to about half past eleven, wakes up and walks her dog, and then winds up watching a late-night movie because she, of course, cannot fall asleep after that evening nap. She has developed "learned" insomnia. Other predisposing factors are physical health problems, particularly those causing chronic pain; heavy caffeine and/or alcohol use; poor sleep habits; a history of psychological problems, such as depression, anxiety, and somatization disorders (recurring, chronic physical ailments, such as gastrointestinal pain, without physiological basis); and the inclination to habitually internalize emotional conflicts.

Precipitating Factors

Precipitating factors are the events that set off your sleep problems. Understanding what started your sleep difficulties can help determine the treatment strategy. Examples of precipitating factors are: dosage and timing of a new medication, a stressful life event (e.g., marriage, childbirth, death or illness of loved one, or work- or school-related stress), the onset of a physical illness or injury, a change in environment (e.g., move to new home or travel to an unfamiliar place), and a change in diet.

Perpetuating Factors

These are factors that cause insomnia to continue, often developing after the insomnia symptoms begin. The original cause of your sleep problem may have subsided, but certain factors are causing the sleep disturbance to continue. Below is a list of factors that commonly perpetuate insomnia (Spielman and Glovinsky 1997):

* spending too much time in bed

* irregular sleep-wake schedule

* ongoing worry that lack of sleep will interfere with daytime responsibilities

* napping, dozing during the day

* intermittent sleep

* caffeine consumption

* alcohol or drug consumption

* learned, reinforced behaviors

Assessing Your Sleep

Although situational or transient insomnia often resolves spontane-ously, you must recognize that it can also represent the beginning of a longer-term problem. Therefore, early identification and interven-tion (professional and/or self-help) play a crucial role in prevention of a more chronic problem. This can be accomplished by paying attention to precipitating factors (see above), and by taking a look at your maladaptive sleep behaviors—negative ways in which you might think, feel, or behave around your sleep-wake habits. In this section, I present ways in which you will be able to evaluate the extent of your own sleep disturbance. I recommend that you look at the following areas: circumstances surrounding the start of your sleep difficulties; severity and frequency of your sleep problems; daytime consequences of your sleep difficulties; what treatments have been helpful or not helpful in the past; and factors that improve or aggra-vate your symptoms (e.g., other medical problems, use of medications, current emotional concerns, work issues, and/or family issues).

First, it will be helpful to take a personal history of your sleep. Read the list of questions below, think them over, and jot down your answers. If you wish, share them with a family member or close friend and bring any concerns to the attention of your physician or other health-care provider (Lacks 1987).

1. How many nights per week do you have difficulty falling asleep?

2. How many minutes does it take for you to fall asleep after going to bed, particularly on the nights that you have some difficulty?

3. Do you ever wake up in the middle of the night? How many nights per week? On average, how many times do you wake up each night? How many minutes does it take you to get back to sleep each time?

4. How often do you wake up early in the morning, before your scheduled wake time, and are not able to fall back to sleep?

5. On the nights when you seem to have insomnia, about how long do you sleep during the night?

6. How long have you had a sleep problem?

7. How long would you like to sleep each night?

8. Is your sleep problem sometimes worse than it is at other times?

9. Why do you believe you have a sleep problem?

10. Was the onset of your symptoms related to any specific event?

11. What do you do when you cannot sleep?

12. When you try to sleep, is it difficult to turn off your mind and thoughts?

13. Have you experienced more stress than usual lately?

14. How often is your sleep interrupted by environmental factors, such as traffic, neighbors, and family members?

15. How dark is your bedroom at night? Could it be made darker?

16. How many times per week do you nap?

17. Do you engage in regular exercise? How often?

18. How many caffeinated beverages do you drink in a day? How many do you drink after four o'clock in the afternoon (e.g., coffee, tea, or cola)?

19. Do you use any other drugs, such as alcohol, allergy medications, pain medications, or nicotine?

20. Does your difficulty sleeping ever influence your mood or ability to function during the day?

21. Do you snore or ever wake up unable to breathe?

22. Do your legs ever jerk repeatedly or feel restless after you go to bed at night?

23. Do you work a night, rotating, or split shift?

24. Do you have any physical problems or illnesses, such as headaches, gastrointestinal problems, or pain from an injury?

25. What, if any, self-help remedies have you tried for your sleeping problems?

Answering these questions will help you understand your sleep patterns in general, as well as your feelings about your sleep problems.

Next, try keeping a daily sleep diary for a least a week. Keeping a sleep diary are is an important part of assessing your own sleep difficulties. I have included a sample diary in appendix B. As you will see, the sleep diary asks you to record information regarding naps, how long it takes you to fall asleep, number and duration of night wakings, total sleep, and quality of sleep. The purpose of a sleep diary is to continuously monitor your insomnia and/or other sleep problems. If you keep a sleep diary for approximately a week, your own data will give you a better sense of whether you are satisfied with your sleep and/or any changes you could make to improve or lessen your sleep difficulties.

These self-assessment tools will provide you with valuable baseline information regarding the intensity of your symptoms. After you have made some changes in your sleep-wake habits, you may want to make use of the diary or the questions above in order to appraise your improvement and (I hope) pat yourself on the back for your hard work. On the other hand, self-reporting can be biased, since some of us are likely to exaggerate our symptoms or deny or be oblivious to our sleep disorder. If you have any questions or do not find helpful the interventions suggested in the next section, it is crucial that you contact your physician, health-care provider, psychologist, or local sleep-disorders clinic for advice regarding your sleep problem.

Preventing and Managing Your Insomnia

Current treatments for insomnia depend upon the cause and duration of the problem. Transient and intermittent insomnia may not require intervention since episodes last only a few days at a time. For example, if your insomnia is due to a temporary change in your sleep/wake schedule, as with jet lag (and I sure had a terrible case of jet lag when we traveled east to Israel a few summers ago), your - circadian clock will often get back to normal on its own. However, if you experience daytime sleepiness and impaired performance at work or in caring for your children, the use of short-acting sleeping pills may improve your sleep tonight and your alertness tomorrow. For example, a friend and colleague of mine described her personal experience with transient insomnia:

My first bout with insomnia came early in my pregnancy. I did not know exactly what caused my sleep difficulties. One thing I am sure of is that I wasn't physically uncomfortable due to weight gain, because I had only gained about five pounds at the time my symptoms started. The insomnia would probably have lasted longer if I had not discovered that Benadryl [antihistamine] is safe to take during pregnancy. [Of course, if you are pregnant, check with your own physician before taking any medication.] I had the same insomnia symptoms at the beginning of my second pregnancy. I could fall asleep at the drop of a hat during the day, but if I did that, it made the nights even more torturous. It seemed that I could fall asleep fine, but inevitable I would wake up a few hours later unless I took Benadryl. So, I was resigned to taking the medication for a very brief period to prevent the development of more chronic and severe insomnia.

However, as with all drugs, there are potential side effects. The use of over-the-counter sleep medicines is not usually recommended for the treatment of insomnia. Whatever the cause, it is always suggested that sufferers of insomnia keep a sleep diary (discussed above) in order to document both the pattern of their insomnia and the effectiveness of various treatments as they are introduced.

Treatment for chronic insomnia is done in four steps. First, any underlying medical or psychological problems are often diagnosed and treated. However, this is not always necessary. Increasingly, research and clinical practice suggests that it may be important to simultaneously treat insomnia and the underlying medical or emotional condition, as opposed to ignoring the insomnia while treating the primary problem. Second, it is important to identify behaviors that may worsen the insomnia and try to stop or reduce such behaviors or habits. Third, medications are often used to treat the insomnia. In the National Sleep Foundation's *Sleep in America Poll* (2000), approximately one-fourth of adults said that they have taken medication to help them sleep in the past year. Nearly twice as many women (30 percent) as men (17 percent) reported that they use medications to help them sleep. Of those adults who used a sleeping medication, over 50 percent used over-the-counter medications, 35 percent used prescription medications, and 10 percent used both. Fourth, a variety of behavioral approaches are used for healing chronic insomnia. In the next section, I present a number of behavioral approaches involving actions you can take to improve your sleep. Combining behavioral and medical approaches may be helpful for some women.

Cognitive Behavioral Practices Used for Treating Insomnia

Behavioral techniques may prove to be helpful either in reducing the risk of insomnia, or even in preventing it altogether. In fact, psychologists have shown that nonmedical therapies produce reliable and long-lasting benefits for people with insomnia who have trouble falling and staying asleep (Morin, Culbert, and Schwartz 1994). The techniques or treatments range from limiting the time spent in bed (sleep restriction) to making a stronger mental connection between bed and sleep. This latter approach is called stimulus control. Studies suggest that these two strategies are the most effective cognitive-behavioral approaches (Morin, Culbert, and Schwartz 1994). Other behavioral approaches include, sleep hygiene and relaxation therapy. Many people find that using a combination of the recommended techniques is most beneficial. For example, Dr. Jack

Edinger and his colleagues recently demonstrated that cognitive behavioral therapy (e.g., sleep education, stimulus control, and sleep restriction) produces greater improvement for chronic primary insomnia in comparison to relaxation therapy alone or a placebo (Edinger, Wohlgemuth, Radtke, Marsh, and Quillian 2001). You may want to ask a sleep specialist (e.g., psychologist, social worker, physician, or nurse) to help you use these strategies properly and most effectively. In the paragraphs that follow, I outline the cognitive-behavioral techniques that are most efficacious for your insomnia. These are the Sleep-Smart Strategies for this chapter.

Sleep Hygiene

This approach involves countering behaviors that interfere with sleep—focusing on your health practices or habits (e.g., diet, exercise, and substance use) and environmental factors (e.g., light, noise, and temperature) that affect your sleep. Often sleep hygiene education also involves acquiring basic information regarding sleep and changes in sleep patterns over the course of one's life. In the section below, I describe some of the behaviors that are important to resist because they may interfere with your sleep, which by now should be very familiar to you.

1. Avoid heavy meals before bedtime. If necessary, have a light snack before bed (mainly starch, some protein, and a warm drink).

2. Avoid strenuous exercise within two to three hours of sleep. You will find that regular exercise earlier in the day helps sleep.

3. Avoid tobacco, alcohol, and caffeine. Alcohol may assist with falling asleep, but it disrupts overall sleep patterns.

Relaxation Therapy

This technique is also helpful for improving sleep, particularly for those who suffer from insomnia. A number of studies indicate that relaxation procedures can produce improved sleep (Lichstein and Riedel 1994). Specific techniques can be effective in decreasing and/or eliminating anxiety and body tension. If you experience difficulty falling asleep and/or falling back to sleep during the night, you may feel like your mind is racing and your muscles are tense. Relaxation techniques should help you slow your racing thoughts and relax your muscles so that you experience a more restful, calm sleep. See appendix B for more detailed instructions regarding relaxation strategies.

Counting practices are probably the best-known method to relax a person to sleep (my parents certainly told me to count those sheep many times). Here's one counting exercise to try:

Take a slow, deep breath. Allow your muscles to relax. Try not to resist the thoughts that come into your mind, but try not to follow them, either. Instead, go with them and give yourself an alternative focus. Notice as the thoughts float into your consciousness ... then observe them as they float away. Notice your breathing. Count an inhale as one, an exhale as two, and so on. When you reach five or ten, go back to one. Relax your breathing. Breathe as slowly and deeply as you comfortably can. There does not need to be any strain—only calmness and appreciation that you can rest now after all of the day's activity. You can also try counting a succession of visualized objects (such as the stereotypical flock of sheep jumping one by one over a fence), but counting breaths has an advantage: they are real, and you probably will not feel as silly as you might when tracking those imaginary sheep.

Here is another technique that you can call upon to help you relax:

1. Assume a comfortable posture.

2. Clear your mind by stopping disturbing thoughts.

3. Tune out distractions by concentrating on breathing, sensations, a sound, a phrase, or a scene.

4. Combine deep relaxation with verbal training (e.g., tapes), pleasant visual images, relaxing bodily sensations, such as warmth or heaviness, or meditation.

5. Practice, practice, practice your relaxation exercise on a daily basis (fifteen minutes, two times per day).

Stimulus Control

This therapy consists of a set of instructional procedures designed to curtail sleep-incompatible behaviors and to regulate your sleep-wake schedule. If you have insomnia, the steps in this therapy are meant to help you recondition yourself to associate bed and bedtime with sleep. You may have come to associate bed and bedtime not with sleeping, but with being awake and unable to sleep, with negative thoughts and feelings about sleep, and with doing non-sleep activities in bed (e.g., doing office work, watching television, talking on the phone, or paying bills). With this particular healing process, you will try to learn to reassociate your bed and bedroom with rapid sleep onset. The bed and bedroom will not be as strongly associated with other activities. You will learn to maximize the cues that are associated with feeling sleepy and falling asleep, and to decrease the cues that you associate with staying awake. The following instructions are the basic steps of this relearning process (Bootzin, Epstein, and Wood 1991; Lacks 1987):

1. Use your bed and bedroom only for sleep (and sexual activity).

2. Go to bed and lie down only when you are sleepy.

3. Establish a regular presleep routine, and make your sleep environment quiet, dark, and comfortable in temperature.

4. When you get into bed, turn out the lights for sleep. If you cannot fall asleep after about ten to fifteen minutes, get up and go to another room. Choose a quiet, relaxing activity to do until you feel drowsy, such as reading a boring magazine or listening to soothing music (do not read the latest spine-tingling thriller!)

5. Repeat step 4 as often as necessary until you fall asleep, and if you awaken during the night.

6. In general, avoid naps, and go to bed and wake up at the same time each day, regardless of how much sleep you got during the night. This will help your body to attain a consistent sleep rhythm.

Sleep Restriction

This approach is another highly recommended behavioral therapy method intended to help you regularize your sleep and wake patterns (Spielman, Saskin, and Thorpy 1987). Sleep restriction therapy consists of limiting the amount of time spent in bed. Those who suffer from insomnia may spend too much time in bed unsuccessfully trying to sleep. For example, if you report sleeping an average of five hours out of eight or nine hours spent in bed per night, the initial prescribed sleep window (i.e., from initial bedtime to final rising time) would be five hours.

The allowable time in bed is increased or decreased by fifteen to twenty minutes (or kept stable) for a given week depending on whether one's sleep efficiency (i.e., the proportion of the night spent actually asleep) that week increases, decreases, or remains the same (Morin, Culbert, and Schwartz 1994). Adjustments are made periodically until an optimal sleep duration is achieved. You may benefit from a sleep restriction program that at first allows only a few hours of sleep during the night, and gradually increases your time to sleep until you achieve a more normal and efficient night's sleep. Below are recommended steps for the sleep restriction approach:

1. Try to avoid naps during the day.

2. Define your optimal sleep length (i.e., the amount of sleep you need in order to feel good during the day).

3. Set your alarm and get up at the same time every morning, no matter how much sleep you got during the night.

4. Go to bed at a time that is consistent with your current sleep duration (even if it is short) and get up at a set time. When you are able to sleep 95 percent of that duration, you may begin to lengthen your sleep time by about fifteen to twenty minutes (i.e., go to bed 20 minutes earlier). When sleep is 95 percent of the lengthened time, repeat these steps until you reach your optimal total sleep time.

Cognitive Therapy

Many people have a number of misconceptions or beliefs about sleep that actually hinder their ability to sleep. (I hope that I have been able to dispel some of *your* sleep myths.) One cognitive-behavioral approach to ending insomnia is to learn to get rid of such incorrect beliefs and to replace them with appropriate and helpful interpretations. Psychologists refer to this approach as cognitive therapy. Charles Morin (1993) described five types of dysfunctional cognitions, or unhelpful thoughts and beliefs, that may be familiar to those who experience insomnia:

1. misconceptions about the causes of insomnia;

2. misattributions regarding the consequences of poor sleep;

3. unrealistic sleep expectations;

4. decreased perceptions of control and predictability of sleep; and

5. faulty beliefs about sleep- promotion habits. Let's take a look at some of these common dysfunctional sleep thoughts and some suggestions for changing such inappropriate beliefs.

You may have thought at one time or another that your never-ending insomnia can damage your physical well-being. However, there is no evidence that anyone has ever died from lack of sleep alone. Moreover, worrying too much about your insomnia may simply make your insomnia worse.

Another common dysfunctional belief is that it's necessary to get eight hours of sleep every single night. This is an unrealistic expectation. As discussed earlier, sleep needs vary widely among adults. If you tend to experience insomnia, try to avoid placing too much pressure on yourself to achieve such high sleep standards. Again, such pressure may actually increase your anxiety and maintain the insomnia. (And, if you are not an insomniac but perhaps tend to skimp on sleep, don't believe the myth that one can thrive on just a few hours of sleep. While sleep needs differ by the individual, studies on alertness have shown that even with as much as six or seven hours of sleep per night, some weakened alertness does occur. And most of us are poor at judging our own level of alertness accurately.)

I have heard some of my friends say, "When I do not get an adequate amount of sleep, I have to catch up by sleeping late the next day or by napping." This misconception, that it is necessary and possible to make up for sleep loss, is very common. Unfortunately, it isn't really possible to make up for lost sleep and, in fact, oversleeping in the morning or taking daytime naps may delay the onset of your sleep the next night. Sleep researchers recommend that you only need to recoup about one-third of your previous night's sleep loss.

Another common dysfunctional belief is that all of us have the same sleep schedules and patterns. For example, you may assume that because your partner falls asleep in minutes you should be able to do the same. But beyond some general standards, there is variability in how long it takes each of us to fall asleep, how often we wake up during the night, and the duration of our sleep. I recommend that you avoid making comparisons to other people, because they only create more worries and anxieties about your sleep or other aspects of your life (e.g., height, weight, clothing, or career).

Although I cannot possibly include all of the sleep beliefs that are harmful to our sleep-wake patterns, I will discuss one more before moving on: the belief that insomnia is the result of some sort of biochemical imbalance. Regardless of the initial causes, psychological and behavioral factors are usually involved in maintaining chronic insomnia.

Medications Used for Treating Insomnia

I must state my biases up front before addressing this topic: it is my belief, based on research, that cognitive-behavioral treatments for insomnia are most effective, particularly in the long run, for treating the more chronic sorts of insomnia. Increasingly more research is being devoted to evaluating the effectiveness of combining behavioral and pharmacological approaches (Morin, Colecchi, Stone, Sood, and Brink 1995). However, 25 percent of Americans take some sort of medication every year to help them with their sleep (National Sleep Foundation 2000, *Sleep in America Poll*; Shader, Greenblatt, and Balter 1991). If you are struggling with insomnia, consult with your physician to find out whether medication is an appropriate method of treatment for you. And even if your doctor does prescribe a drug to help you sleep, for persistent insomnia, medications should not be the main form of treatment but should be used as adjuncts to a primary behavioral treatment method, such as cognitive-behavioral therapy (Edinger, Wohlgemuth, Radtke, Marsh, and Quillian 2001).

You may believe that sleeping medications that you purchase at the pharmacy, or ask your physician to prescribe, are necessary for sleep. However, some studies actually demonstrate that believing that a sleeping pill has helped with a good night's sleep is the reason the pill is effective, rather than any effects of the pill itself. Additionally, nearly all sleeping medications lose effectiveness if used for a longer period than recommended.

Generally, medications may be taken when: sleep difficulties seem to be interfering with daily activities, insomnia is temporary or short term, when insomnia occurs in association with a diagnosed medical condition, or when behavioral approaches are clearly ineffective. In addition, it is recommended that treatment with medications begin with the lowest effective dose, be used for a short period of time if taken nightly, be used on an intermittent basis, if taken for a long period of time, and be used in combination with good sleep-hygiene practices and/or a variety of behavioral approaches. In the section that follows, I will summarize the various medications that are used for treating insomnia.

Hypnotics

Over the years, as a result of extensive research, it has become clear that prescription medications that promote sleep, called *hypnotics*, are the most effective sleep aids available. Yet, I cannot emphasize enough that the specific medication prescribed by your health-care provider for your insomnia should depend on your symptoms, medical condition, use of alcohol or other drugs, and age.

Benzodiazepines, a particular type of hypnotic, are the preferred drug for treating insomnia (Bliwise 1991). Developed in the 1960s, they are considered safe and effective at promoting sleep. These medications work by acting in areas of the brain believed to be involved in sleep enhancement. Benzodiazepines tend to increase stage 2 sleep but reduce stage 3 and stage 4 sleep, which is considered to be the most restorative. You need stage 3 and stage 4 sleep in order to renew your body. While you may not be growing anymore, during stages 3 and 4 growth hormones are released that help your body heal and refresh for the next day. Stage 2 is the least necessary stage of sleep; it tends to be left out when a person finally sleeps after a period of sleep deprivation.

Hypnotics differ by half-life (i.e., how long a drug is active in the body) and biochemical structure. Drugs with shorter half-lives are recommended so that functioning is not impaired the next day. You may have experienced that terrible feeling of waking up in the morning and feeling drugged and unable to function—this is not how you want to feel after taking any sort of medication. In particular, the benzodiazepine triazolam has a short half-life, as do two non-benzodiazepines, zolpidem and zalephon. Most benzodiazepines have sedative and hypnotic properties, but only five are marketed as hypnotics (see below). All five reduce the time that it takes to fall asleep, decrease the number and duration of night wakings, and increase total sleep time and sleep efficiency, with various degrees of effectiveness. Most are effective with short-term use (four weeks is the recommended limit); minimal data is available on their long-term efficacy. In fact, most sleep specialists emphasize that sleep aids should not be seen as a long-term solution to insomnia.

In general, problems associated with use of hypnotics include: alteration of sleep stages, residual effects residual effects from the drug the following day, return of insomnia symptoms, memory difficulties, dependence on the drug, cognitive and psychomotor impairment (e.g., falling when trying to walk to the bathroom at night), and drug "hangovers." Benzodiazepines are contraindicated for: pregnant women, substance abusers, sleep-apnea patients, individuals who may be called on to preform duties at night, and individuals with depression. Rebound from use tends to be associated with increased anxiety as well as the person's belief that he or she cannot sleep without medication.

Below is a list of the five benzodiazepines and their descriptions:

* Estazolam (ProSom): Newer drug. Takes effect quickly and is less likely than other drugs to remain in the system after awakening; can remain effective for up to six weeks of nightly use. The average reduction in the time that it takes to fall asleep is modest.

* Flurazepam (Dalmane): Accumulates with use; effective in both inducing and maintaining sleep for up to one month of nightly use.

* Quazepam (Doral): Newer drug. Similar to flurazepam, effective for the management of sleep-onset and sleep-maintenance insomnia. It produces less impairment of daytime functioning than flurazepam and its long half-life minimizes the return of insomnia symptoms.

* Temazepam (Restoril): Better for sleep-maintenance than sleep-onset problems and may produce fewest daytime residual effects. Minimal tolerance has been reported for up to three months of use. Probably the best hypnotic for older adults.

* Triazolam (Halcion): Reduces sleep-onset latency; increases total sleep time, with less daytime sleepiness. However, early-morning awakening and daytime anxiety has been associated with use. It has been withdrawn from market in several European countries.

Several nonbenzodiazepine hypnotics are currently used in the United States; some are under development or available in other countries. One of these is zolpidem (Ambien), which has a rapid onset and short duration. It is effective in decreasing sleep-onset latency but is not effective in decreasing either the number or duration of awakenings during the night. As with other short-acting hypnotics, there is evidence of rebound insomnia upon withdrawal.

If you become dependent on benzodiazepines, your dependence may be both psychological and physical in nature. Tolerance to the drug develops, causing the therapeutic dosage to no longer work; as a result you may want to increase the dosage, or keep using the drug even though it is not working. Because insomnia increases temporarily upon ceasing use of benzodiazepines, women (and men) may give up trying to quit using the drug. If you have been taking benzodiazepines, be aware that insomnia will return for a little while as you stop using that drug. If you've been on an intermittent schedule (meaning you take it as needed) you are likely to be more reliant on the drug, even if you do not take them every night, because problematic behavior are more likely to increase when inconsistently reinforced. Before you begin one of the behavioral approaches presented earlier in this chapter, you will want to begin to taper off of your medication. Ask your health-care provider to help you taper your use of benzodiazepines. Below are some guidelines that I suggest you discuss with your health-care provider:

* Set goals for your withdrawal.

* Develop, with the advice of your health-care provider, a week-by-week schedule for tapering off. Some hypnotics require tapering at the rate of one therapeutic dose per week.

* Begin to understand that taking a drug to combat sleeplessness is not as helpful as you think.

* Learn about withdrawal and rebound symptoms. Be honest with yourself about your motivation to discontinue use. If you do not want to stop, it will be harder to stop.

* Introduce drug-free nights. Schedule certain nights during which you do not use any sleeping medication at all. Weekend nights (or non-work nights) are the best times to start.

* Seek therapy from a psychologist or other qualified counselor who can help you deal with emotional aspects of withdrawal and work with you on behavioral techniques for decreasing your insomnia difficulties. As I emphasized earlier, research has shown that behavioral treatment is effective when one either withdraws from hypnotics or maintains a consistent dose of the hypnotic throughout the behavioral treatment (Bootzin and Rider 1997; Epsie, Brooks, and Lindsay 1989).

Over-the-Counter Sleep Medications

Many women use sleep medications that are available without a prescription, called *over-the-counter* (OTC) medications. You certainly can purchase such sleep aids without a prescription; however, OTC medications are often less effective than prescription medications and they are not as thoroughly researched. Examples of nonprescription sleep aids include: Nytol, Sominex, antihistamines, and some pain relievers. Although many have sedating effects, antihistamines are designed to alleviate cold or allergy symptoms, not to promote sleep. As with hypnotics, OTC sleep aids should not be used if you are also taking alcohol or other sedating drugs. Likewise, I recommend that older adults; individuals with breathing difficulties, glaucoma, or urination problems; and pregnant or nursing women avoid these nonprescription medications.

Drugs That Promote Insomnia

Anyone who is trying to eliminate their insomnia should have a clear understanding of the effects of alcohol, caffeine, and other drugs that tend to promote and perpetuate insomnia-like symptoms. So let's examine these drugs and their effects.

Although women and men have consumed caffeinated foods and beverages for hundreds of years, questions persist regarding its effects on women's health. Researchers have investigated the impact of caffeine on women's health, from reproduction to osteoporosis (International Food Information Council Foundation 1998). However, caffeine consumed in moderation produces no adverse health effects. The most commonly known sources of caffeine are coffee beans, cocoa beans, cola nuts, and tea leaves. The amount of caffeine in food products varies depending on the serving size, the type of product, and the preparation method. With teas and coffees, the plant variety also affects caffeine content. Surveys show that caffeine consumption patterns have not changed significantly over the last decade. Average caffeine consumption per person is around two hundred milligrams per day, with pregnant women consuming less caffeine than the general population.

Caffeine is a mild central-nervous-system stimulant. Since caffeine does not accumulate in the body over the course of time, it is normally excreted within several hours of consumption. A brewed cup of coffee contains 100 to 150 milligrams of caffeine, a twelve-ounce can of cola has 40 to 60 milligrams, and a chocolate bar has as much as 20 milligrams per ounce (see caffeine content chart below). For the most part, caffeine increases alertness, delays sleep onset, reduces total sleep time, and increases light (stage 1) sleep, once you have consumed approximately 100 to 400 milligrams (Roehrs 1993). Nicotine, another stimulant, also increases sleep latency and reduces total sleep time and Rapid Eye Movement (REM) sleep (Phillips and Danner 1995). Caffeine's influence in adults lasts about three to five hours, but some people may experience the effects for as long as ten hours. If you experience insomnia, I highly recommend that you cut down on caffeine use in general; if you must have that cappuccino or latte, try to limit your coffee drinking to the morning hours. When regular caffeine consumption is abruptly stopped, you may experience withdrawal symptoms, such as headaches, fatigue, or drowsiness. These effects are usually temporary, lasting for a few days, and often can be avoided if caffeine cessation is gradual. Overall, you will need to find your own acceptable level of caffeine consumption so that it doesn't interfere with your sleep.

Central-nervous-system depressants, such as alcohol, also have profound effects on sleep and wakefulness. It is worth noting that far more studies on the use of alcohol in connection to sleep have been conducted with male participants than with female participants. However, a few studies have questioned older women regarding their use of alcohol to overcome sleep problems. For example, one researcher found that 91 out of 130 women in her sample regularly had wine or a mixed drink before bedtime to promote sleep, and 43 percent of the women who used alcohol also used an OTC medication each night (Johnson 1994, 1997). It appears that alcohol use for its sedative effects is quite common.

It is popularly believed that a drink before bedtime can aid falling asleep. But alcoholic beverages consumed at bedtime, after an initial stimulating effect, may decrease the time it takes to fall asleep. Because of alcohol's sedating effect, many women with insomnia consume alcohol to promote sleep (I can still remember my grandmother's small sherry glass on her nightstand). However, alcohol consumed within an hour of bedtime appears to disrupt the second half of the sleep period (Roehrs and Roth 1997). You may sleep restlessly during the second half of sleep, awaken from your dreams, and return to sleep with considerable difficulty. With habitual consumption just before bedtime, alcohol's sleep-inducing effect may decrease, while its disruptive effects may continue or increase (Vitiello 1997). This sleep disruption may lead to daytime fatigue and sleepiness. Older women and men are at particular risk, because they achieve higher levels of alcohol in the blood and brain than do younger persons after consuming the same amount of alcohol.

Many people have wine, beer, and other alcoholic drinks in the late afternoon (at "happy hour" or with dinner) without drinking again during the rest of the evening. Research indicates that a moderate dose of alcohol consumed as much as six hours before bedtime

Caffeine Content

Avoiding or limiting caffeine is highly recommended. Coffee, tea, chocolate, colas, and some medications are all high in this stimulant, which can make some people feel irritable or nervous, interfere with sleep, and contribute to gastrointestinal distress. Caffeine should certainly be avoided five to seven hours before your bedtime. Also, a daily limit of 200 milligrams of caffeine is recommended by the American Medical Association. The caffeine content of various foods is listed below. Of course, these figures can vary according to the product and method of preparation.

Caffeine Content

		Caffeine Content
Per 10-ounce serving:	Coffee, brewed	170–200 mg
	Coffee, decaffeinated, brewed	5–10 mg
	Tea, steeped for 5 minutes or brewed	50–100
	Hot cocoa	5–20
Per 12-ounce serving:	Cola drinks	40–60
	Canned/bottled ice tea	25–35
Per 1-ounce serving:	Milk chocolate	1–15
	Dark chocolate	20
	Bittersweet chocolate	5–35
Per slice	Chocolate cake	20–30

Adapted from R. Duyff, *The American Dietetic Association's Complete Food and Nutrition Guide* (Minneapolis, Minn: Chronimed Publishing, 1996) and from Mary Ellen Copeland, *The Depression Workbook* (Oakland, Calif.: New Harbinger Publications, 1992) can increase wakefulness during the second half of sleep (Roehrs and Roth 2000; Vitiello 1997). Furthermore, the adverse effects of sleep deprivation are increased following alcohol consumption even after the alcohol has passed through the body (e.g., poor performance on a driving simulator) (Roehrs, Zorick, and Roth 2000).

Finally, although there is no doubt that alcohol use and abuse promotes insomnia, it is less clear whether insomnia can lead to alcohol abuse and alcoholism (Roehrs and Roth 1997). The extent to which women and men with insomnia symptoms are drinking in excess to self-treat their sleep problems is not currently known. In order to protect your health, you and your health-care practitioner may want to carefully review your use of alcohol both in relationship to your sleep and in general.

Symptoms Associated with Circadian Rhythm Sleep Disorders

The majority of this chapter focused on insomnia. A small number of women experience symptoms that are similar to insomnia (e.g., sleep-onset struggles), but are in the family of sleep problems called *circadian rhythm sleep disorders*. (See chapter 1 for a discussion on circadian rhythms.) Circadian rhythm disorders are diagnosed when the timing of sleep episodes is out of kilter with the sleep period that is desired or regarded as the societal norm (Zammit 1997). One's sleep episodes are either shifted to an earlier time (phase advanced) or a later time (phase delayed), or the timing of sleep may be irregular. Adolescents, older adults, people who often travel across several time zones, and people who work night shifts are more likely to experience the symptoms of circadian rhythm disorders.

Briefly, *delayed sleep phase syndrome* (DSPS) is characterized by the following: sleep and wake times that are consistently later than desired (falling asleep at two o'clock in the morning when you want to go to sleep three hours earlier, for example); little or no difficulty falling asleep at the later time or maintaining sleep once sleep has begun; tremendous trouble waking up at the desired time in the morning to get to work or school; and inability to advance one's sleep time to an earlier hour. You may have had the most difficulty with DSPS during your adolescent (middle school, high school, and college) years. Women with DSPS differ from those with insomnia in that they usually have an ongoing pattern of sleep phase delay, continuous and undisturbed sleep, and normal amounts of sleep. Intervention may include delaying sleep in two- to three-hour increments for one to two weeks each (going to bed at five o'clock in the morning for one to two weeks, then at eight in the morning for one to two weeks, then eleven in the morning for one to two weeks, and so on), until you are finally going to sleep at the desired time (*chrono-therapy*); resetting your clock with the use of bright, artificial light (*light therapy*); and/or a combination of these two strategies (Zammit 1997).

Light therapy is administered as follows: To phase advance a sleep-wake pattern (move to an earlier time), bright light is administered for up to two hours after the person wakes up and is avoided a few hours prior to bedtime. To phase delay (move to a later time), light is administered for up to two hours before a usual bedtime and avoided at other times (Eastman, Stewart, Mahoney, Liu, and Fogg 1994). If you think that you may be experiencing a circadian rhythm disorder, talk with your health-care provider or local sleep-disorders center regarding the rental or purchase of a light box to use for light therapy. Even after receiving chonotherapy or light therapy, women find that any major variation in their sleep-wake schedule for a day or two resets their clock back in the delayed direction. However, women (and men) who are highly motivated and amenable to using chronotherapy often report elimination of their phase-delay difficulties (Czeisler, Richardson, Coleman, Zimmerman, Moore-Ede, Dement, and Weitzman 1981).

A small number of people, particularly older women, tend to go to bed very early and have an extremely difficult time delaying bedtime; this condition is called *advanced sleep phase syndrome* (ASPS). Consequently, these women are likely to wake up too early in the morning (Zammit 1997). Individuals with ASPS typically fall asleep before nine o'clock at night and awaken between three and five o'clock in the morning. Primary complaints are excessive evening sleepiness and/or early-morning awakenings. Light therapy is quite beneficial for advanced sleep phase complications.

* * * * *

For many women, insomnia and/or delayed sleep phase syndrome are distressing problems, whether they are chronic or crop up intermittently throughout your life. These problems, particularly insomnia, can make you feel helpless, irritable, depressed, and frustrated, not to mention tired. No matter what methods you use to combat your sleep difficulties, be sure to take care of yourself, eat well, reduce stress, follow Sleep-Smart Strategies, and allow for fun in your life.

* 8 *

Sleep Apnea and Other Sleep Disorders

Most women reading this book have probably experienced some sort of disrupted, irregular, or poor sleep at some point in their life. Undoubtedly, occasional disrupted sleep is a common phenomenon. Yet, some people endure chaotic sleep for months or years. It is estimated that 13 to 50 percent of the U.S. population have a diagnosable sleep disorder (Shapiro and Dement 1994). In chapter 7, I discussed insomnia, a sleep disorder characterized by difficulty falling asleep and/or staying asleep. However, you may be struggling with other sleep disorders. Your sleep may become problematic because things happen to your body during sleep (e.g., involuntary leg movements, difficulty breathing) so you wake up feeling tired and unrefreshed, or because you fall asleep during the day at inappropriate times. In this chapter, I review sleep disorders, particularly those that involve excessive daytime sleepiness that many women are confronted with at various times in their lives.

Sleep-Disordered Breathing

Sleep apnea, a type of disordered breathing in sleep, is a condition in which people momentarily stop breathing during sleep. The most common type, *obstructive sleep apnea*, involves repeated complete or partial collapse of the upper airway during sleep. Historically, when women complained of daytime sleepiness and snoring, health-care providers have not automatically thought of sleep apnea, as they ordinarily have done with men. Increasingly more data demonstrates that approximately 25 percent of women over sixty-five have sleep apnea, yet the disorder continues to be under diagnosed (National Sleep Foundation 1998). While sleep apnea is far more common in men, its occurrence increases dramatically in women after age fifty. For example, several recent studies have documented that the risk of sleep-related breathing disorders is almost as high for post-menopausal women not taking hormone replacement as it is for men (see chapter 5). Far more women than previously expected experience breathing disorders related to sleep apnea. Currently, the male-to-female ratio for apnea is about three or four to one, which is quite different from the ten to one ratio usually seen in sleep-disorder clinics (Young, Palta, Dempsey, Skatrud, Weber, and Badr 1993).

All too often, snoring is regarded as humorous and embarrassing when reported or noted in women, rather than as a possible indicator of serious medical problems. In our culture we are likely to visualize the snorer as an overweight man. In fact, the disorder that is now called obstructive sleep apnea syndrome was initially observed by researcher C. Burwell and his colleagues in 1956 in an obese male patient who presented with upper-airway obstruction, snoring, and daytime somnolence. He labeled this the Pickwickian Syndrome, after the character Joe the fat boy in Charles Dickens's novel *The Pickwick Papers*. According to Burwell, Joe the fat boy was a large, somnolent messenger who was portrayed as being extremely sleepy in a variety of situations (Burwell, Robin, Whaley, and Bikelman 1956). This image of the fat boy or man who snores and has sleep apnea has made it difficult for physicians, and women themselves, to consider a possible diagnosis of sleep-disordered breathing in women. Recent research has clearly demonstrated that women's sleep-apnea symptoms do not differ significantly from those of men, and that women show no reluctance to admit that they snore (Young, Palta, Dempsey, Skatrud, Weber, and Badr 1993). Health-care providers, on the other hand, tend to be less likely to thoroughly investigate women's reports of snoring and other related symptoms than they are with men's reports of these symptoms. It is very important that women, with their health-care providers, seek treatment for severe snoring and daytime sleepiness, because sleep apnea and related disorders are linked to automobile accidents, cardiac disease, high blood pressure, stroke, and pregnancy-related hypertension.

Sleep Apnea Defined

So, what exactly is sleep apnea, anyway? It is a breathing disorder characterized by quite brief interruptions of breathing during sleep. The name comes from a Greek term, *apnea* (want of breath).

Snoring is often associated with sleep apnea. However, many snorers do not have apnea and, likewise, some individuals with diagnosed sleep apnea do not snore. At one end of the continuum is snoring unassociated with any breathing disruption. Although (as you may know all too well) simple snoring often poses relationship issues for the snorer's bed partner, it is not a serious health risk for the snorer without any breathing disruption. In fact, you may have even developed insomnia after being awakened by your partner's nightly snoring. But some snoring is associated with intermittent, brief, partial to complete cessations of breathing during sleep. Pulmonologists (physicians who specialize in breathing disorders) define a partial decrease in airflow for ten seconds or more as *hypopnea* (low breathing), and complete cessation of airflow for ten seconds or more as *apnea* (absence of breathing) (Rothenberg 1997).

There are two types of apnea—obstructive and central. Of the two, obstructive sleep apnea (OSA) is far more common. It occurs when the airway collapses, resulting in partial or complete blockage of airflow into or out of a person's nose or mouth, although efforts to breathe continue. As you get into deeper sleep, you stop breathing when the muscles in your airway begin to relax. Then you wake up briefly (but not to full awareness) and the airway opens again. This apnea happens over and over again throughout the night. The airway collapse may be caused by excessive pharyngeal tissue, a large uvula, fatty deposits near the base of the tongue, or the collapse of the pharyngeal walls. In addition, a deviated septum (where the membrane wall between your nostrils is crooked and blocks one side of your nose), enlarged tonsils, or blockage resulting from allergies, colds, sinus infections, and so on may all increase snoring and make sleep-disordered breathing problems worse.

With obstructive sleep apnea, apneas may occur several times to several hundred times during the night, disrupting the progress of sleep from one stage to another. You will notice that as your sleep becomes more fragmented from such awakenings, you experience sleepiness. Without a doubt, excessive daytime sleepiness is one of the hallmarks of severe obstructive sleep apnea. Central sleep apnea occurs when partial or complete cessation of airflow occurs in the absence of any effort to breathe. In this case, the brain fails to send the appropriate signals to the respiration muscles to initiate breathing. Central sleep apnea is sometimes associated with complaints of insomnia as well as daytime sleepiness.

Impact on Women's Lives

Thankfully, sleep apnea is now recognized as a significant health problem. Even mild to moderate cases of sleep-disordered breathing may be associated with strokes, heart attacks, angina (heart-related chest pain), and high blood pressure in both men and women (Fletcher 2000; Young and Peppard 2000). Significant snoring alone, even without sleep apnea, may indicate the presence of cardiovascular disease.

Results from ongoing studies in the near future will greatly increase our knowledge and ability to assess the association between sleep-disordered breathing and cardiovascular disease (Simon, Hsia, Cauley, Richards, Harris, Fong, Barrett-Connor, and Hulley 2001).

In addition to these major health problems, sleep apnea and the sleep deprivation that results from it can also affect the quality of your life in other ways. Individuals with sleep-related breathing problems complain of morning headaches, dry mouth upon awakening, memory loss, attention and problem-solving difficulties, and mood swings (Engleman, Kingshott, Martin, and Douglas 2000). The sleep depravation resulting from sleep apnea can lead to depression, and it may disrupt your professional, family, and social life. Excessive daytime sleepiness from sleep apnea and other sleep problems is not only bothersome, but also dangerous. Individuals with sleep apnea have nearly seven times more automobile accidents than do the rest of the population, and approximately half of the drivers involved in sleep-related accidents have some sort of sleep disorder (George 2000). Sleep researchers and transportation experts report that sleep-related accidents comprise approximately 20 to 40 percent of all vehicle accidents on major roads (Horne and Reyner 1995). It is interesting to note that although sleep-disordered breathing seems to be associated with a higher rate of motor vehicle accidents, this is only true with regard to men drivers (Young, Blustein, Finn, and Palta 1997). More intriguing is the fact that among women there does not seem to be an association between objective measures of sleepiness (see below) and accident rates. Nevertheless, sleep disorders and problems that result in excessive daytime sleepiness may place drivers of both sexes at risk due to their diminished perception of driving conditions, and related factors.

So, what exactly is excessive daytime sleepiness? You may be all too familiar with the feeling that you just cannot stay awake for one more minute (although I hope you don't have this feeling while reading my book!). Sleep clinicians have two main ways to define sleepiness. The first is *subjective sleepiness,* or your own personal sense of how sleepy or alert you are. This method of measuring sleepiness makes a lot of sense to the individual—you—but it is often unreliable because most of us are not good at accurately recognizing our own level of sleepiness versus alertness. For example, many individual with insomnia symptoms describe themselves as very sleepy and yet cannot seem to fall asleep. And, correspondingly those with sleep apnea or other sleep problems that bring on daytime sleepiness often rate themselves as more alert than they actually are.

Objective sleepiness, on the other hand, is determined by observing sleep behavior (Krieger 2000). Objective sleepiness is usually assessed in a sleep laboratory where clinicians or technologists measure the speed with which the individual falls asleep and the actual occurrence of sleep episodes.

Identifying Your Own Sleep-Disordered Breathing Difficulties

Since sleep apnea and related difficulties are often underdiagnosed, particularly in women, below are some clues or signs that may help you to determine whether you are at risk for sleep-disordered breathing (Ancoli-Israel 1996; Orr 1997):

* Your partner mentions that he has noticed that you stop breathing during your sleep.

* Your bed partner has moved out of the room or frequently threatens to do so because your snoring is extremely loud and keeps him up much of the night. Snoring is not always a symptom of apnea. Approximately 25 percent of men and 15 percent of women are habitual snorers, and snoring becomes more common as people age, particularly women.

* Others living in your home (such as your children) hear you snore.

* You feel tired, fatigued, lethargic, or "out of it" in the morning or throughout your day even when you supposedly had a good, long night's sleep.

* You awaken with a headache regularly.

* You have difficulty concentrating or remembering things at work and at home.

* You find yourself falling asleep or fighting to stay awake at inappropriate times throughout your day (e.g., at a meeting, at your child's soccer game, at church or synagogue, while talking to friends, in class, or while working). You have an uncontrollable urge to close your eyes and fall right to sleep.

* While driving, you have nearly caused one or more accidents because you fell asleep or struggled to stay awake while driving.

* You have had a car accident due to falling asleep at the wheel.

Assessing and Treating Your Sleep-Disordered Breathing

If you have any of the symptoms discussed above or you suspect that you have a sleep-related breathing disorder, consult your physician and or an accredited sleep laboratory for an evaluation right away. The American Academy of Sleep Medicine (see appendix

C) can help you locate the nearest accredited sleep center in your area. If you are overweight, you should seriously consider enrolling in a weight-loss program, because weight loss can help reduce obstructive sleep apnea (Saskin 1997). Avoid sleeping medications, alcohol, and other drugs (e.g., morphine, anesthetics, and other similar medications). Sleeping medications and alcohol are respiratory depressants; they make breathing more difficult, make apneas last longer, increase the number of apneas per night, and make it harder to wake up, both in the morning and during the night. Therefore, since an individual with sleep apnea needs to wake up in order to start breathing again, sleeping medications are dangerous for those with sleep-disordered breathing problems (Young, Palta, Dempsey, Skatrud, Weber, and Badr 1993).

Sleep-disordered breathing does not go away on its own—it definitely requires medical treatment from a sleep-disorder clinic. As you work with your physician, you will see that selection of therapy depends on many factors. Below are several sleep smart strategies that you will want to discuss with your physician (adapted from Saskin 1997).

Weight Loss

As mentioned above, many individuals with sleep apnea are overweight. Weight reduction can lead to improvement of your obstructive sleep apnea (Saskin 1997). Perhaps you are stuck in a cycle of despair concerning your difficulty losing weight. Your daytime sleepiness and fatigue may be contributing to your feeling lethargic, unmotivated, and down in the dumps, which, of course, gets in the way of exercising. Although it is difficult to get started on an exercise program, it should be considered as one of the first steps to take in the treatment of your sleep apnea. Discuss an effective diet plan with your health-care provider. He or she may recommend that you work with a team—your physician, a nurse, a dietician, and perhaps a support group. Support groups can be extremely helpful for those who need an extra push, some encouragement, and a bit of TLC in order to get going on a weight-loss program.

Management of Medications

Avoid respiratory suppressant products (e.g., alcohol, sedative medications, and narcotics) if you have or suspect that you have sleep-disordered breathing.

Continuous Positive Airway-Pressure Treatment (CPAP)

The preferred treatment for sleep-disordered breathing at this time is Continuous Positive Airway-Pressure Treatment (CPAP). CPAP does not cure sleep apnea, but it helps keep the airway open during sleep. First introduced in 1981, CPAP involves a high-flow blower that delivers a continuous stream of air into a sealed, relatively comfortable mask that you, the patient, wear over your nose during sleep (Sullivan, Berthon-Jones, Issa, and Evers 1981). The air blower sends positive air pressure through a hose into your nose and airway. The air pressure keeps the airway open while you are sleeping. Your physician or a specially trained technician tests the various air pressure levels while you sleep in the laboratory, to determine which pressure is best for you. Successful use of CPAP is associated with lessening or eliminating most sleep apnea episodes, increasing oxygen, and normalizing your sleep stages. Patients often notice remarkable improvement in their daytime functioning as well. Since you need to wear your CPAP mask every night, manufacturers have developed machines that are portable and can be brought along when traveling.

Dental and Surgical Interventions

A variety of dental appliances have been developed for the management of sleep apnea. Dental orthotic devices are particularly recommended for those who experience primary snoring or who have mild to moderate sleep apnea (Schmidt-Nowara, Meade, and Hays 1991). Consult your physician and/or dentist to determine whether these devices are appropriate for you.

Finally, surgical interventions may be used in certain cases of sleep apnea. In surgery the airway is enlarged by tightening the flabby muscles in the airway, removing unnecessary tissue, and shortening the uvula. Although surgery often eliminates snoring, it only helps sleep-disordered breathing in some people, some of the time. Research is under way to improve surgical treatment for sleep apnea and related disorders.

Let's now move on to a discussion of other disorders that may affect your sleep.

Periodic Limb Movements Disorder and Restless Legs Syndrome

Periodic Limb Movement Disorder (PLMD) is a condition that is characterized by the jerking of the leg (or arm) during sleep (Montplaisir, Nicolas, Godbout, and Walters 2000). Each twitch may last from .5 to 5 seconds, occurring about every 20–40 seconds. They may occur over a period of a few minutes or several hours. In severe cases, the twitches may continue all night. The movements themselves do not pose any health risk, and some of you may experience them without any problems. However, if the twitches are strong, or if you are a light sleeper, they disturb your sleep and wake you up.

When you awaken, you will not know what disturbed you. Over time, these frequent awakenings are likely to result in excessive daytime sleepiness. Some women experience PLMD during pregnancy (see chapter 3). To date, researchers have not determined the specific cause of these movements; however, PLMD is related to certain medications, poor circulation, a metabolic disease, kidney disease, or folic acid deficiency.

Women with PLMD often complain of sleep-onset insomnia; as soon as they relax enough to fall asleep, their legs begin to twitch and jerk, waking them up again. Obviously, if you have trouble falling asleep or wake up numerous times during the night due to these leg and/or arm jerks, you are likely to feel exhausted and excessively sleepy during the day. On average, individuals with PLMD sleep approximately an hour less each night than those without PLMD. Often this disorder goes undiagnosed, which is what happened to one of my friends and colleagues:

> It took two years for doctors to figure out that I have a sleep disorder. One winter when I was in my late twenties, I experienced extreme fatigue, weakness, daytime sleepiness, headaches, and other debilitating symptoms. I'd had mononucleosis seven years earlier, so my doctor thought I might have been reinfected or be experiencing a chronic type of mono. I was tested for Lyme disease, thyroid disorders, and numerous other conditions, all of which turned up negative. Eventually I was diagnosed as having chronic fatigue syndrome and was left to struggle with that on my own. For the next two years, I was disabled by fatigue. There were days when I'd wake up after sleeping for twelve hours, take a shower, and be so exhausted that I immediately had to go back to bed. I was so weak and tired that I had to sit on the floor to blow-dry my hair—I didn't have enough energy to stand and hold my arms over my head at the same time! I could not concentrate on my work, had memory difficulties, and could not process information properly. It seemed as if I was working in slow motion while everyone else sped around me. I could only work about four hours a day, and then I had to go home and sleep. I felt like I had a brain injury. Furthermore, I experienced all sorts of physical symptoms such as headaches, nausea, digestive problems, allergies, and food sensitivities, and I lost a significant amount of weight. Two years later, I changed doctors, and my new doctor sent me for a sleep study. He thought I might have sleep apnea, because I had reported waking in the middle of the night, feeling like I was gasping for air. He was on the right track, but he had the wrong disorder. I was diagnosed

with Periodic Limb Movements Disorder (PLMD). Although I was not aware of it, during my sleep I was experiencing severe "twitches" or "spasms" that would cause my legs to kick out and awaken me from the deeper levels of sleep. Although the diagnosis of this condition focuses on leg movements, I know that I also experience these "spasms" in my back, neck, and shoulders. As a result, I was spending about 80 percent of my sleep time in Stage 1 and Stage 2 sleep, and only about 10 percent of my sleep time in REM sleep. I was severely Rapid Eye Movement (REM) deprived, which is what was causing many of my symptoms. Once I was diagnosed and treatment started, I felt an improvement almost immediately. I knew that we had found the culprit because none of the other treatments that I had tried in the last two years had worked, but this one did. Slowly, I returned to normal functioning, although it took two years to gain back all the weight that I had lost. I know that I will always have this disorder. I've noticed that its severity fluctuates with my menstrual cycle (it's worse in the week immediately before my period begins) and, of course, it's worse when I'm stressed. I still experience chronic sleep deprivation and feel more fatigued than the average person, but I've learned how to manage the disorder. In addition to medical treatment, I have to adhere to good sleep hygiene principles. So far, it's been working and I've gone from being someone who could barely work four hours a day to being a successful college professor who works more hours each week than she should!

Many women (and men) with PLMD also have Restless Legs Syndrome (RLS), and almost all of those with RLS have PLMD (Montplaisir, Nicolas, Godbout, and Walters 2000). With RLS, strong sensations are felt deep within the thigh, leg muscles, knees, or even ankles that cause a powerful urge to move the leg. Some individuals also feel these sensations in their arms. Women have explained to me that it feels like bugs crawling, or a creeping, crawling, tingling, pulling, and/or painful sensation, occurring when the person lies down or sits for a long period of time, such as when working at a desk, riding in a car, watching a movie, or listening to music. Women with RLS also describe an irresistible urge to move their legs when the sensations occur. Moving the legs, walking, rubbing or massaging the legs, or doing knee bends can bring relief, at least briefly. RLS symptoms tend to follow a daily cycle, becoming more bothersome during the evening and night hours. RLS sufferers may find it difficult to relax and fall asleep because of this strong urge to walk or do other activities to relieve the sensations in their legs. Similar to sleep apnea and PLMD sufferers, those with RLS may feel extremely sleepy during the day. The severity of symptoms varies from night to night and over time. Some individuals may find that they have periods when RLS stops causing problems, but the symptoms usually return. Below is a list of the common characteristics of RLS:

* Unpleasant creeping, crawling, tingling, pulling, or painful sensations are felt in the legs and sometimes in the arms.

* Relief of leg sensations occurs with walking, stretching, knee bends, massage, or hot or cold baths.

* Leg discomfort occurs when lying down or sitting for long periods of time.

* Symptoms worsen in the evening and during the night.

* Involuntary leg (and occasionally arm) movements occur during sleep (PLMD).

* Falling asleep or staying asleep is difficult.

* Sleepiness or fatigue is experienced during the day.

* Family members have similar symptoms.

Restless Legs Syndrome seems to occur in both women and men. Symptoms may start at any time but tend to be more common and more severe with age, often during the third decade in life. Young girls who experience symptoms of RLS are sometimes misdiagnosed with "growing pains" or considered hyperactive because they cannot sit still in school. Although the cause is unknown in most cases, certain factors seem to be associated with RLS and PLMD:

* Family history. Often RLS and PLMD run in families, so women whose mothers had one of these syndromes may be likely to develop one or both symptoms themselves.

* Pregnancy. Some women experience RLS during pregnancy, especially in the last months, but the symptoms usually disappear after delivery (see chapter 3).

* Low iron levels or anemia. Women with these conditions may be prone to develop RLS; the symptoms may improve once the iron level or anemia is corrected.

* Chronic diseases. Kidney failure quite often leads to RLS. Other chronic diseases such as diabetes and rheumatoid arthritis may also be associated with RLS.

* Caffeine intake. Decreasing caffeine use may improve symptoms.

* Alcohol use. The likelihood of having a "clinically significant" number of periodic leg movements (more than twenty per hour of sleep) and symptoms of RLS is three times more in women who consume two or more alcoholic drinks each day than in those who drink fewer than two drinks per day (Aldrich and Shipley 1993).

RLS can be difficult to diagnose. No laboratory test can make a diagnosis of RLS, and when you initially consult a physician, he or she will probably not be able to see anything obviously wrong with you. Diagnosis, therefore, depends on your detailed description of your symptoms to your doctor (who may in turn recommend that you see a neurologist). Your partner may be able to help by describing how your leg movements awaken you. A complete physical and neurological exam will help identify other conditions associated with RLS, such as nerve damage. Basic laboratory tests may be conducted in order to assess general health and to rule out anemia. Finally, your physician may suggest that you undergo an overnight sleep study to determine whether PLMD or other sleep problems may be contributing to your sleep difficulties. All in all, RLS can be a very frustrating sort of sleep problem to pin down. However, health-care providers are becoming more adept at making early diagnoses and sleep researchers are developing and evaluating new treatments.

The mother of one of my students shared her experience of RLS with my research team:

> When I was about thirty-seven, I began to get annoying, strange, tingling feelings in my legs occasionally when I would sit down at the end of a tiring day. Sometimes it would happen when I was seated on an airplane, and often it happened as soon as I sat in a car. Most frequently, though, it would happen at night when I went to bed. The sensation of bugs crawling in my legs would wake me up three or four times a night. In my efforts to deal with the constant need to move my legs I would often take up to eight extra-strength pain relievers per night. At the time the symptoms started, I was a full-time working mother. I did not initially attribute the lack of sleep I was getting to the uncomfortable feelings in my legs. I was usually tired at work and I thought I might be suffering from chronic fatigue syndrome. When I asked my doctor about my symptoms, she realized that I had restless legs syndrome.
>
> Ten years later, now at age forty-seven, I am still battling restless legs syndrome. The symptoms still arise when I am tired or have been on my feet for a long time. Since seeking professional medical help, though, I have begun to manage my RLS differently than before. I have found that if I have my legs

massaged or sit in a hot tub at the end of the day, my leg muscles seem to stay more relaxed during the night. A prescription medication used by Parkinson's disease patients, Sinemet, has also aided in relieving my symptoms. Also, I am currently looking into certain exercises and natural vitamins that may reduce the severity of restless legs. Overall, today I am able to live more comfortably and sleep more soundly with daily RLS treatment.

So, how are RLS and PLMD treated? In mild cases of RLS, some people find that certain activities, such as taking a hot bath, massaging the legs, using a heating pad or ice pack, exercising, and eliminating caffeine, help alleviate symptoms. In a more severe case, your health-care provider may prescribe medication to control symptoms. Unfortunately, no one drug is effective for everyone with RLS. Individual women respond differently to medications depending on the severity of their symptoms, other medical conditions, and other medications they are taking. A medication that is initially effective may lose its effectiveness with nightly use; so it may be necessary to rotate medications to keep symptoms under control. Although many different drugs may help with RLS, three types of medications (see below) are most commonly used below (Montplaisir, Nicolas, Godbout, and Walters 2000). Discuss these medications with your physician to find out which may be best for you.

* Benzodiazepines, such as Klonopin or Restoril, are central-nervous-system depressants that do not fully suppress RLS sensations or leg movements but allow you to obtain more sleep despite these problems. These medications reduce the number of awakenings at night, but they have little effect on the number of actual leg jerks. In other words, you still kick your legs, but you do not tend to awaken as often.

* Dopaminergic agents are drugs used to treat Parkinson's disease; they are also effective for those with RLS and PLMD. These medications have been shown to reduce RLS symptoms and nighttime leg movements.

* Opioids (e.g., Tylenol with codeine) are painkillers and relaxants that suppress RLS and PLMD in some people. These medications reduce the number of leg kicks, but they do not always decrease the number of awakenings. Moreover, opioids are potentially addictive and should be used at the lowest possible dose and, like all prescription medications, should be taken only if prescribed by your physician.

For more information on RLS, contact the Restless Legs Syndrome Foundation, Inc. (see Resources).

Narcolepsy

Narcolepsy, the most dramatic intrusion of sleep into one's waking life, is yet another sleep disorder that presents with excessive daytime sleepiness. It is estimated that two to five persons in a thousand have this rather debilitating disorder (Webb 1992). As Marguerite Jones Utley (1995) explained in her book, *Narcolepsy: A Funny Disorder That's No Laughing Matter,* "narcolepsy is a strange, odd, weird disorder." Narcolepsy is a neurological sleep disorder that is experienced by both women and men that causes persistent and excessive daytime sleepiness (similar to sleep apnea). Yet, it is easily distinguished from other sleep disorders because it is characterized by episodes of cataplexy, a sudden loss of muscle control. Unfortunately, this disorder is often misdiagnosed as fatigue, depression, or some other form of mental illness. Sufferers typically experience symptoms for a decade or longer before the disorder is diagnosed. Narcolepsy is not curable, but it is not fatal, either, although its symptoms may result in serious or fatal accidents.

The absolute cause of human narcolepsy is still unknown. However, recent research suggests that narcolepsy involves an interaction between environmental factors (e.g., abrupt change in sleep-wake schedule and/or severe personal stress) and specific genes (Mignot 2000). More than 85 percent of all individuals with narcolepsy who suffer from cataplexy share a specific genetic marker (Guilleminault and Anagnos 2000). A second gene involved in narcolepsy has been located in narcoleptic dogs and mice (Mignot 2000). These discoveries may eventually lead to changes in the approach to the diagnosis and treatment of narcolepsy and related sleep disorders.

The individual who suffers from narcolepsy experiences the following symptoms:

* Excessive daytime sleepiness, often with brief, recurring, uncontrollable sleep episodes or *sleep attacks* during waking time;

* Cataplexy—sudden, brief loss of muscle control, usually triggered by emotions such as laughter, anger, fear, or surprise, while the person remains conscious;

* Hypnagogic hallucinations—vivid, realistic, often frightening dreams that occur while the person is falling asleep or waking up;

* Sleep paralysis—partial or total paralysis of voluntary muscles when going to sleep or waking up; and

* Disrupted nighttime sleep, in which the person wakes up many times during the night for a variety of often unexplained reasons, possibly dreams among them.

For the most part, narcolepsy is treated with medications, prescribed by a physician (usually a neurologist), and scheduled naps. The goal of treatment is to keep the person with narcolepsy awake and able to function during the day using the minimal effective dose of medication. The commonly prescribed medications include: central-nervous-system stimulants (such as Ritalin), antidepressants, sedatives, and hypnotics. If you suspect that you may have narcolepsy, please contact your physician as soon as possible.

*   *   *   *   *

As you have read, sleep disorders and problems with sleep may be brief, intermittent, and/or chronic. Ambiguous symptoms, lack of knowledge on the part of health-care professionals, and symptoms being mistaken for signals of a variety of other emotional and/or physical health problems may mean that your sleep problems go unrecognized. For this reason, it is important that you advocate for yourself when seeking help from health-care providers. If you suspect that you have a sleep disorder, speak up and ask for help; if your health-care provider doesn't have sufficient knowledge in this field, ask for a referral to a specialist or sleep-disorder clinic. Insomnia and excessive daytime sleepiness are the most common sleep-related reasons for women to seek professional help. Since these sleep difficulties, along with SDB, RLS, and PLMD, often affect your ability to feel good about your work and home responsibilities, your emotional well-being, and your physical health, appropriate assessment and treatment is important to pursue. Undoubtedly, professional help for your sleep disorder will significantly improve your quality of life.

Sleep problems can indeed affect our physical and emotional well-being. However, our physical and/or emotional well-being can influence our sleep-wake patterns. In the following chapter, I discuss physical health problems and their relationship to sleep.

* 9 *

Physical Health and Sleep

Last night was a rough night for me—I slept terribly. I did not have trouble falling asleep, but at around two o'clock in the morning I was awakened by stomach discomfort, a sinus headache, and other aches and pains. I was not able to fall back to sleep for nearly two hours. I just could not get comfortable, and I tossed and turned trying to fall back to sleep. After a while, I finally got up and took some ibuprofen for my headache. Then, I got back in bed and, although I was now slightly more comfortable in the physical sense, all of my worries about the next day started to race through my mind. It was very stressful! Fortunately for me, however, I have few of these trying nights. But, for many women, my difficulties would probably seem small in comparison to some of their sleepless nights.

In this chapter I explore the intricate relationship between sleep disturbances and women's physical well-being. Several health problems are more prevalent in women, including fibromyalgia and migraines. The pain associated with these disorders often interferes with sleep. Below, I discuss fibromyalgia, headaches, and other related health problems that bring pain and discomfort that often interfere with our sleep patterns. I offer Sleep-Smart Strategies for improving your sleep in the face of these chronic conditions; you may find that these strategies can also be applied to other health problems that involve chronic or intermittent pain and discomfort.

Fibromyalgia

Fibromyalgia, also called fibromyalgia syndrome (FMS), is a complex, chronic condition that causes generalized pain and fatigue, along with a variety of other symptoms. Unlike arthritis, fibromyalgia does not cause pain or swelling in the joints themselves; rather, it produces pain in the soft tissues located around joints, skin, and organs throughout the body, known as tender points. Fibromyalgia is often referred to as the "irritable everything syndrome" or the "invisible disability," because the symptoms are not easily identifiable (St. Amand and Marek 1999; National Fibromyalgia Partnership, Inc. 1999). It is estimated that up to 10 million Americans (2 to 4 percent) suffer from fibromyalgia, with 90 percent of adult cases occurring in women (Wolfe 1993). Onset of fibromyalgia usually takes place between the ages of twenty-four and sixty-five.

Fibromyalgia is not a new illness, although awareness of it has grown rapidly in recent years. In Victorian times, it was known as neurasthenia. More recently, it was referred to as fibrositis, a misnomer, because the suffix -itis suggests inflammation.

The cause of fibromyalgia is not currently known, but recent research has revealed that the illness often develops following a physical trauma (i.e., accident, injury, or severe illness) or is associated with an infection (Goldenberg 1993). Researchers have found that fibromyalgia was thirteen times more likely to occur following a neck injury than following an injury to lower extremities (Buskilia, Neumann, Vaisberg, Alkalay, and Wolfe 1997). On the other hand, not everyone with fibromyalgia experienced an obvious physical trauma prior to the onset of symptoms. Other research suggests a familial pattern, with fibromyalgia more common on the female side of the family (Donaldson, Buskila, Neumann, Hazanov, and Carmi 1996).

So what are the symptoms associated with this troublesome but yet not crippling or fatal illness?

Symptoms

In addition to pain and fatigue, those with fibromyalgia may report one or more of the following (St. Amand and Marek 1999; Wolfe, Hawley, Cathey, Caro, and Russell 1985):

* Stiffness—aching pain and stiffness in muscles, tendons, and ligaments. Often this stiffness is worst at rise time and after prolonged periods of sitting or standing in one position. Stiffness may occur during changes in temperature or humidity.

* Headaches and facial pain—migraine, tension, or vascular headaches. Some FMS sufferers experience headache pain in the temples and/or behind their eyes. Also, many women (and men) with fibromyalgia experience pain in the temporomandibular joint (TMJ) area (where the jaw meets the ear).

* Gastrointestinal—irritable bowel symptoms, including gas, pain, bloating, alternating constipation and diarrhea, and sometimes nausea.

* Genito-urinary problems—increased urgency or need to urinate, with or without a bladder infection. Some women also have more painful menstrual periods or increased fibromyalgia symptoms during menstruation, vaginal spasms or cramps, and other related symptoms.

* Skin complaints—itchy, dry, or blotchy skin; rashes; occasional swollen, hot itching palms and soles of feet; and the sensation of something crawling under the skin. Some individuals also experience a sensation of swelling in the fingers and toes. In addition, persons with fibromyalgia tend to be sensitive to temperature; similar to people with Raynaud's Syndrome, some individuals have an unusual sensitivity to cold in their hands and/or feet, which is accompanied by color changes in the skin.

* Cognitive and emotional changes—often, women with fibromyalgia are misdiagnosed with depression and/or anxiety disorders. Fibromyalgia is neither a form of depression nor an anxiety disorder, symptoms of depression and/or anxiety disorders may coexist with fibromyalgia. In particular, many women experience fatigue, irritability, nervousness, depressed mood, difficulty concentrating, and/or memory difficulties. These symptoms are experienced upon awaking in the morning.

* Sleep disturbances—although many women with fibromyalgia get an adequate amount of sleep, they are likely to report that they awaken feeling unrefreshed, as if they had barely slept. Others may have trouble falling or staying asleep (similar to insomnia; see chapter 7). The reasons for this nonrestorative sleep and the other sleep difficulties that tend to accompany fibromyalgia are basically unknown. However, recent research is beginning to make some sense of the sleep problems that coexist with fibromyalgia. I will discuss sleep and fibromyalgia later in this chapter.

Sleep and Fibromyalgia

Clinical studies show that more than 75 percent of patients with fibromyalgia complain of poor sleep (Wolfe 1993). Those in this group describe their sleep as light, unrefreshing, and accompanied by generalized stiffness, aching, and profound fatigue upon awakening in the morning (Moldofsky, Scarisbrick, England, and Smythe 1975). Individuals with fibromyalgia and coexisting poor sleep seem to experience more pain, physical disability, and emotional distress in comparison to those without sleep difficulties. It is clear that disturbed sleep is a significant component of the disabling features of fibromyalgia (Moldofsky 1995).

In particular, the majority of individuals with fibromyalgia also have an associated sleep disorder known as alpha-EEG anomaly. In this disorder, the individual's deep sleep (stages 3 and 4) periods are interrupted by bouts of waking-type brain activity. As a result of this anomaly, those with fibromyalgia tend to wake up feeling tired, worn out, and in pain. Moreover, individuals with fibromyalgia tend to have reduced REM sleep and increased non-REM sleep. Some women (and men) with fibromyalgia experience fragmented sleep also as a result of periodic leg movements, sleep apnea, bruxism (grinding the teeth), and *sleep myoclonus* (a sudden rapid contraction of a muscle or a group of muscles during sleep or as one is falling asleep).

One of my colleagues, who runs a group for fibromyalgia sufferers, shared her concerns regarding fibromyalgia and sleep:

> My fibromyalgia patients are always exhausted. Many of them are convinced that they never get any slow-wave sleep. They will wake up at the slightest noise and often stay fully awake and alert for hours after. Some of the women (and 99 percent of my clients are women) have a mix of sleep-onset insomnia [difficult falling asleep] and sleep-maintenance insomnia [difficulty staying asleep]. One patient actually has sleep-onset insomnia due to pain. She not only has fibromyalgia, but she also suffers from osteoarthritis, rheumatoid arthritis, and degeneration of the joints.
>
> The majority of my clients are all too eager to use medication in an attempt to help them sleep better. The most popular is amitriptyline, but others include Restoril, Paxil, and Tylenol PM. The idea of using sleep-management strategies often causes frustration and skepticism in these women. Cutting back on caffeine, forming a wind-down bedtime ritual, and exercising can help substantially. I spend entire sessions of therapy on sleep, because understanding sleep is the first step to improving one's own sleep quality. Unfortunately, many individuals I work with are just in too much pain to try new sleep schedules or practices.

Undoubtedly, sleep disturbances may be responsible, in part, for the low energy levels and muscle pain experienced by many - people with fibromyalgia. And, of course, this nasty combination of pain and fatigue often limits physical activity and endurance. In one study, women with fibromyalgia recorded their sleep quality and pain intensity for thirty days. The researchers found that the women who reported poor sleep also reported higher pain levels. Additionally, a night of poor sleep was followed by more daytime pain, and a more painful day was followed by a night of even poorer sleep—a vicious cycle of poor sleep and pain.

Interventions for Fibromyalgia

Individuals are most likely to see significant improvement in their pain symptoms and daytime functioning if their fibromyalgia symptoms are identified early and they are highly motivated to do what they can to feel better (St. Amand and Marek 1999). Therefore, if you suspect that you have fibromyalgia, it is crucial that you discuss your concerns with your health-care provider and seek out resources (see appendix C) that will be helpful to you. Research suggests that effective treatment for fibromyalgia must take a multifaceted approach focusing on pain reduction, correcting posture, stretching and exercise, stress reduction, improving sleep habits, and (sometimes) use of medications (St. Amand and Marek 1999).

Below are some of the interventions for fibromyalgia. Although many of the recommendations may seem to have little to do with sleep, they may be beneficial to your sleep in the long run by helping to decrease pain and discomfort and thereby enabling you to sleep more efficiently.

* Physical Rehabilitation. Ask your health-care provider to refer you to a physical therapist. The most widely used physical therapy techniques for fibromyalgia are massage; myofascial release (a therapy designed to relieve restrictions and tightness in connective tissue); trigger point therapy (a technique focusing on hyperactive spots in the muscles where the nervous system is overly active); stretching; and postural training.

* Aerobic Exercise. Practiced with the advice of a physical therapist and/or physician, daily gentle, low-impact aerobic exercise is often quite beneficial to people with FMS (McCain, Bell, Mai, and Halliday 1988). It helps prevent muscle atrophy by promoting blood circulation to the muscles and connective tissues, and it improves strength and endurance. Examples include walking, doing warm-water exercise, swimming, using treadmills, and cycling. Avoid exercising the most painful muscles, and begin any new exercise program slowly in order to avoid injury and build strength in increments. Exercise produces the best sleep benefits in the late afternoon or early evening. If you find that your exercising increases your pain or creates new pain, stop immediately and consult your physician and/or physical rehabilitation therapist.

* Occupational Therapy. Some job-related responsibilities, tasks, or environment contribute to fibromyalgia pain, such as performing repetitive movements, or sitting in uncomfortable chairs or work stations. If this is the case for you, I recommend that you consult an occupational therapist who can help by suggesting or designing improvements.

* Relaxation Therapy. Effective stress management is important for all of us and it is particularly important for those with fibromyalgia. Not surprisingly, your pain and related symptoms may bring on stress, and this stress may in turn exacerbate your fibromyalgia symptoms. Often, breathing exercises, progressive muscle relaxation (PMR), and guided imagery are useful for reducing symptoms of fibromyalgia. (See the relaxation exercises in chapter 7 and appendix B.) However, women with acute pain (e.g., from fibromyalgia, endometriosis, migraines, or severe backaches) might not want to try PMR because it involves tensing one's muscles and therefore could exacerbate discomfort or pain in the most affected areas (Domar and Dreher 1996). If you do want to try PMR, you may want to try tensing and relaxing muscles in the parts of your body that are not causing you extreme discomfort. Generally speaking, use good judgment and common sense in order to protect your health.

* Cognitive or Behavioral Therapy. Attitude, thinking patterns, and motivation are often the strongest predictors of how well you will be able to manage your fibromyalgia or other chronic health condition. Research suggests that individuals who are not actively taking charge of their illness, who feel like victims, and who become helpless are less likely to see improvement. Consulting a psychologist or other mental health practitioner specializing in cognitive/behavioral therapy may be beneficial; she may be able to help you manage your symptoms, guide you to decrease your "learned helplessness" behaviors, teach you to change your negative thinking patterns, and encourage you to schedule pleasant activities that can act as distracters from your chronic or intermittent pain. Also, consider keeping a pain diary (see appendix B), in order to determine just how bad the pain really is—your negative perceptions of your pain may be making it seem worse than it is.

* Medications. It is crucial for you to consult a health-care provider with expertise in treating fibromyalgia so you can be sure that you are making use of the most effective medications available. However, there is no magic pill for fibromyalgia. Medications that are effective with FMS appear to work mainly by increasing sleep time and eliminating disruptions in Stages 3 and 4 sleep (Goldenberg, Felson, and Dinerman 1986). Amitriptyline (Elavil)

and cyclobenzaprine (Flexeril) are the most commonly prescribed and helpful to individuals with fibromyalgia. Sometimes, non-steroidal anti-inflammatory drugs (NSAIDs) are helpful for acute pain relief. For more information regarding medical treatment of FMS, please consult your physician.

* Sleep Habits. Getting adequate sleep is important for all of us, and it is essential for people with fibromyalgia. FMS symptoms often appear during times of sleep disruption, which may be due to stress, night-shift work, pain from an injury, or having to get up to attend to young children during the night. Since sleep is so important for reducing fibromyalgia symptoms, you should create a relaxing sleep environment with a comfortable mattress and room temperature, and no noise, lights, or disruptive pets in the room. Avoid late-evening liquids, alcohol, caffeine, and heavy foods. During the day, take a brief nap, even if it is just for thirty to sixty minutes. At times, re-establishing your regular sleep schedule may be enough to provide relief from your symptoms. If you are tired at night, *go to bed*—set your alarm for half an hour earlier than usual and do those unfinished tasks in the morning. (Your responsibilities will still be there in the morning, and you will find that they take far less time if you deal with them when you are rested and not sleep deprived.) Finally, you may find it helpful to keep a sleep-wake diary (see appendix B).

Most women with fibromyalgia can be helped by using a combination of therapies—maintenance of a regular sleep schedule, exercise, physical therapy, stress management, and often medication. If you are experiencing any of the symptoms discussed above (e.g., chronic aching, pain, stiffness, tender muscles, headaches, or excessive daytime sleepiness), share this information with your physician or health-care provider so that you can receive the appropriate treatments.

Like fibromyalgia, chronic headaches can also interfere with sleep. In the next section, I describe the different types of headaches and their relationship to sleep.

Headaches

Headaches are a very common problem—over 90 percent of individuals experience them at some time during their lives. The majority of headaches last for a very short time. For example, a headache associated with a virus improves when the illness has run its course; headaches associated with skipping a meal or two go away within a few hours. With these sorts of headaches, the underlying cause is usually readily apparent to the sufferer.

Other headaches, however, do not have an obvious explanation, and they may lead to considerable worry and anxiety for the sufferer. These unexplained headaches are referred to as *benign recurring headaches,* accounting for approximately 75 percent of headaches. These ordinary headaches, sometimes referred to as tension headaches, may be brought on by stress, noise, prolonged concentration, eyestrain, or drinking too much alcohol. Benign recurring headaches are considered a widespread minor health problem.

Many women (including myself) suffer from a more serious form of headaches, migraines. Migraines are three times more common in women than in men (Stewart, Lipton, Chee, Sawyer, and Silverstein 2000). In a sample of fifteen hundred U.S. households, 6 percent of men and 18 percent of women reported having one or more migraine headaches each year (Stewart, Lipton, Celantano, and Reed 1992). Migraine headaches appear in women primarily from puberty through menopause, with an average prevalence of 25 to 30 percent during this time. In general, during the young adult and middle years, headache complaints in women outnumber those of men about three to one. At this time, the literature on the relationship between headaches (migraines and others) and sleep or lack of sleep is minimal.

Migraine Headaches

A migraine headache is defined as an episodic headache lasting from four to seventy-two hours and associated with nausea and/or vomiting (Goldmann and Horowitz 2000). In between migraine headaches, most individuals have no symptoms, yet may experience other headaches, such as tension HAs. Daily headaches are not migraines. Symptoms of migraine include: headache, visual disturbances, aversion to light, nausea, vomiting, aversion to food, and lethargy. Some migraine attacks are preceded by visual disturbances (aura). Migraine headaches usually ease within twenty-four hours of starting, but they can last anywhere from a few hours to three days. The frequency of attacks varies; on average, migraines are experienced about one to two times per month, but a small number of women may suffer from migraines once or twice a week. At times, several months or years may pass between migraines, for no apparent reason. In general, attacks become less frequent after age fifty-five.

Although health-care providers do not know why we get migraine headaches, certain factors seem to trigger attacks. Not every trigger will automatically bring on a migraine, yet usually more than one factor is involved. In the section below, I discuss the common trigger factors and some recommendations for eliminating or minimizing such triggers.

* Sleep-pattern changes: Getting too little sleep may be problematic and trigger migraines and other headaches for some women. Others may notice the onset of a headache after sleeping late, even a mere thirty minutes longer than usual, or while lying in bed dozing—typically on a weekend morning, just when you are taking a moment to relax. Maintaining a regular sleep-wake schedule has many benefits, including preventing or decreasing migraines for some women.

* Specific foods: Cheese, chocolate, citrus fruits, alcohol (particularly red wine), coffee and tea (both consumption and withdrawal from these), and sweets may trigger a migraine, although how these triggers work is unknown. If you think that a particular food or beverage is precipitating your migraines, eliminate that food from your diet for approximately two months to see if this diet change decreases your migraines. Keep a headache diary to carefully record any changes (See Migraine and Tension Headache Assessment in appendix B). If the frequency or intensity of your migraines does not change, reinstate the food and eliminate another possible trigger food for two months. It is recommended that you make such diet changes under the guidance of your health-care provider.

* Insufficient food: Delaying or skipping meals or eating too little food may lead to a migraine. (I myself am guilty of missing meals when I get too busy.) Some women find that they can control the timing of their migraines by eating small, nutritious snacks at frequent intervals throughout the day.

* Medications: Oral contraceptives and other drugs that constrict or dilate blood vessels, such as nitrates. If you are on oral contraceptives (birth-control pills) and you experience migraines, it is recommended that you consult your physician.

* Emotional events: For some women stress and anxiety may trigger migraine and other headaches Other women may feel fine when under stress but find that migraines begin just when they have a moment to relax. Unfortunately, stress is unavoidable in our lives, but it is important to recognize its signals in ourselves and find techniques for coping with stress, since it can affect our sleep, emotions, and physical well-being.

* Environmental factors: Bright or flickering lights, weather or temperature changes (e.g., increased humidity), strong smells, loud noises, and changes in altitude can all bring on migraines.

* Hormonal changes: Pregnancy, taking oral contraception or HRT, and menstruation can trigger migraines. Read on for more information on hormones and migraines.

Hormone-Related Headaches

The striking connection between migraines and menstruation was actually first recorded by Hippocrates in the fifth century B.C.E. (Goldmann and Horowitz 2000). For several centuries following, physicians believed that the *womb* was to blame for headaches. Thankfully, physicians and researchers now understand the complex relationship between migraines, hormones, and the brain. An area of the brain, the hypothalamus, operates the menstrual cycle's complex control system, sending messages to the ovaries and the uterus. Therefore, it is actually the brain that initiates hormone-related headaches.

Researchers have found that 50 to 60 percent of women who experience migraine headaches have more headaches before and during menstruation than they do at other times during the month (Rains and Sheftell 2000). In particular, 10 to 14 percent of these women note that their migraines occur around the time of their period and rarely at other times, and approximately 15 percent report that they experienced their first migraine in the same year in which they menstruated for the first time. Researchers and clinicians refer to such migraines as *menstrual migraines*. So-called menstrual migraines occur in the two days before a period and during the first three days of bleeding, and at no other time during the month. Such migraines seem to be connected to the decrease in estrogen that occurs during the menstrual cycle (see chapter 2). If you experience menstrual migraines, you may also notice that changing hormone levels also affect your response to other migraine triggers. For example, you may be more susceptible to the effects of red wine and other alcoholic drinks, sleep deprivation, and skipped meals at this point in your menstrual cycle.

Some women may also experience increased migraines while taking oral contraception, during pregnancy, and during menopause. Most migraine sufferers who take oral contraceptives do not notice any changes in their headaches. Moreover, most physicians argue that it is safe for women who experience migraines to take oral contraceptives unless their migraine symptoms include an aura (Goldmann and Horowitz 2000). Recently developed oral contraceptives contain much lower doses of estrogen than the earlier versions did and, therefore, the overall risk of thrombosis (blood clotting) is extremely low in healthy, nonsmoking women, under age forty. Nonetheless, if you experience migraines and would like to use oral contraceptives, discuss your migraine history in detail with your health-care provider, so you can be sure to maintain your good health.

The relationship between migraines and pregnancy is unclear. Some women notice that their migraines diminish or seem less severe during the second and third trimesters of pregnancy, whereas others experience no changes. On occasion, women have their first migraine attack while pregnant or their migraines may begin to include an aura. Following childbirth, you may experience migraines due to interrupted and decreased sleep, but migraines also often return with the restart of menstruation. In a recent study of first-time mothers (assessed at the time of childbirth and at five and twelve months thereafter), the largest group (one-third of the women surveyed) reported having had migraines, sleep problems, and depressed mood at one year postpartum (the time when many women resume menstruation) than they had earlier in the year (Saurel-Cubizolles, Romito, Lelong, and Ancel 2000).

The largest group of individuals who seek advice regarding migraines are women in their early to mid-forties. During the perimenopausal years, the ovaries produce decreasing amounts of estrogen, which seems to lead to more frequent and more severe migraine headaches (see chapter 5). These hormone changes, as well as the sleep loss that comes with night sweats, can trigger an increase in migraines. Although some women continue to experience migraines following menopause, migraines decrease or disappear for many at this time. Yet, in the general population over age sixty, the incidence of migraines in women is twice that in men (Rains and Sheftell 2000). This statistic suggests that some factors other than hormones contribute to the predominance of migraines in women; however, further research is required.

Many menopausal women use hormone replacement therapy (HRT) to treat the symptoms of menopause (see chapter 5). Few studies have evaluated the effect of HRT on migraines, however. Like any hormone changes, oral contraceptives, and other medications involving hormones, HRT may aggravate migraines in some women but lead to improvement in others. If you have a history of migraines and are considering HRT, be sure that your health-care practitioner knows about your migraines and that you discuss the various options with him or her. Of course, not all headaches are migraines. Below is a discussion of other types of headaches and what may cause them.

Tension and Other Headaches

Nonmigraine headaches may be related to stress, lack of sleep, eyestrain, certain drugs, sinusitis, hypertension, or a head or neck injury. A tension headache is defined as a pain or sensation of tightness, pressure, or constriction that varies in intensity, frequency, and duration; these headaches seem to affect the entire head, as opposed to just one side as is common in migraines. Those who experience tension headaches may feel that the pain never recedes and occurs nearly every day. These headaches are likely to throb in the early morning and develop into a dull ache during the day. If you suffer from these headaches you may notice signs of tension in your muscles, such as tense jaws or clenched hands. Often, such headaches occur in anticipation of, during, or following recognizable stressful situations. Major life events, such as marriage, the birth of a child, the loss of a parent, and career changes all can contribute to stress. However, research suggests that it is day-to-day stress or chronic hassles that are likely to trigger tension headaches. It is important to identify such stressors or hassles early so that you can prevent or diminish the severity of tension headaches, because they can interfere with daytime functioning as well as nighttime sleep. Below are some of the most common stresses:

* Multiple-role stress: Many of us overextend ourselves trying to play several roles at once—mother, partner, working woman, volunteer, caregiver for aging parents. Try to avoid this stress by scheduling time to nap, to sleep at night, and to relax. You may find it helpful to actually make an appointment for yourself to relax, nap, or go to bed, and *show up on time* for this special appointment. Should someone at work or home ask you to do something during that time, respond by saying, "I have an appointment," or "I am busy at that time." Making your rest a priority will help you deal with everyday stress and make you less susceptible to tension and migraine headaches.

* Workplace stress: As discussed in chapter 6, the majority of women in the United States today work outside the home. In addition, although increasingly more women hold high-status positions, most of us have jobs that place high demands on us but offer us little control. These sorts of positions may lead some women to feel helpless in their work environment at times. Feelings of helplessness can worsen the physical and emotional effects of stress and may prevent you from working to improve your situation. Such stress and negative emotions may provoke the onset of tension headaches. To combat those helpless feelings, try to incorporate activities into your life that make you feel good and give you back a sense of control—get to the gym on a regular basis, cook your favorite healthy meals, and make time every day to read from a good book, for example. The time you take for yourself will help you regain your perspective.

* Financial stress: Women, on average, earn less money and have a lower standard of living than men do, and over one-quarter of woman-headed households are poor, particularly minority

households (U.S. Census Bureau 1999). As a result, many women feel pressures as a result of inadequate housing, poor access to health care, challenges of getting and paying for child care, and ongoing worries over making ends meed. With these pressures, it may be difficult to avoid daily stress. Yet, whenever possible, try to find that moment for yourself, so that you can have the strength to stand up to these difficulties.

* Depressed and/or anxious feelings: Headaches are not psychological problems, and the majority of headache sufferers do not have significant psychological difficulties. However, headache sufferers tend to have increased daily stress or more difficulty coping with stress and, therefore, often report symptoms of depression and/or anxiety. Moreover, if you are feeling depressed and/or anxious, your headaches may be made worse by these feelings, which in turn may be made worse by sleep difficulties. In chapter 10, I discuss at length the relationship between sleep complaints, depression, and anxiety disorders.

Sleep and Headaches

Not a lot of literature regarding the connection between sleep (or the lack of sleep) and headaches is available. Physicians are only beginning to query their patients regarding their sleep habits when they present with headache symptoms, much less during routine office visits. It behooves you as the patient to be proactive and emphasize your sleep concerns to your health-care provider, since sleep disorders may contribute to headaches and pain from headaches may exacerbate sleep difficulties, such as insomnia. Specifically, migraine attacks may be precipitated by sleep deprivation, but excessive sleep is also sometimes associated with migraines (Inamorato, Minatti-Hannuch, and Zukerman 1993). However, in the majority of situations where sleep is a factor, migraines are precipitated by sleep deprivation and relieved when the sufferer falls asleep.

Other researchers and clinicians are focusing on morning headaches and sleep disorders, particularly obstructive sleep apnea (OSA) and periodic leg movements in sleep (PLMS) (see chapter 8). In a recent study of patients with either OSA or PLMS, 60 percent reported having had headaches in the year prior to the study, and nearly 50 percent reported having had headaches upon awakening (Loh, Dinner, Foldvary, Skobieranda, and Yew 1999). Morning headaches were significantly more common in those with OSA than those with PLMS. Brief (shorter than thirty minutes) morning headaches seem to be associated with OSA, and their occurrence and severity increase with the severity of the OSA. Research suggests, however, that morning headaches improve when OSA patients make use of Continuous Positive Airway-pressure Treatment (CPAP; see chapter 8).

Preventive Approaches and Interventions for Headaches

According to the American College of Physicians, nearly 70 percent of those with migraines have tried some sort of alternative to drug treatment for their migraines (Goldmann and Horowitz 2000). The following nonmedical treatments are most helpful in reducing the effects of triggers:

* Physical therapy. This form of treatment may reduce neck and back pain, which can trigger migraines, and it also increases relaxation. Licensed physical therapists work in conjunction with physicians, nurses, and other health-care providers.

* Osteopathy and chiropractic care. Like physical therapy, osteopathy and chiropractic care may reduce the pain in the back, neck, legs, and other areas that can trigger migraines. This medical field focuses on problems relating to bones and muscles.

* Acupuncture and acupressure. Some migraine sufferers find that using these two treatments helps to prevent attacks. Pressing on tender points during an attack can bring relief.

* Massage. Regular use of massage can reduce tension in the muscles and minimize headaches resulting from stress. Your local health club may offer inexpensive massage services to its members.

* Yoga and exercise. Yoga stretches muscles, relieves stress, helps with breathing, and eases tension. Many health clubs and fitness centers offer classes in yoga, and you can teach yourself other relaxation strategies through the use of video- and audiotapes. Massage, yoga, and exercise all reduce the effects of migraine triggers, but they are not necessarily helpful once the migraine has started.

Medical or drug treatments are also often necessary for migraine sufferers. A number of medications can be used to prevent migraines and/or reduce the pain once you have a full-blown migraine. Consult your health-care provider to discuss the medical options that are right for you. A wide range of different prescription medications are used to either prevent or decrease the number of migraines, or to control the severity of the attack, such as ergotamine, triptans, antidepressants (e.g., amitriptyline and nortriptyline), beta blockers (e.g., metoprolol and propranolol), valproate sodium (not suitable for pregnant women), and calcium channel blockers. If it appears that relief from headache pain is requiring increasingly higher doses of over-the-counter or prescription pain medication, please discuss these *rebound headaches* with your healthcare provider. Several studies have pointed out that misuse or over use of painkillers (e.g., aspirin), ergotamines, or triptans can result in the return of the headache as the medication wears off. The warning signs include chronic early-morning headaches, steady increase in the effective dose, and worsening of the headache several hours after taking a dose of pain medication. A combination of nonmedical strategies and medication may be beneficial for women who experience chronic migraines and/or tension headaches. In particular, in decreasing triggers and the occurrence of headaches, you may find that your sleep improves as well.

*   *   *   *   *

Physical health problems such as fibromyalgia and headaches, which involve chronic or intermittent pain, can intensify sleep difficulties and contribute to daytime sleepiness. Although this chapter is focused on fibromyalgia and headaches, a variety of other health problems can contribute to pain and as a result interfere with sleep. Some of these health problems or illnesses include premenstrual syndrome, endometriosis (both discussed briefly in chapter 2), thyroid problems, and chronic back pain. It is my hope that some of the intervention strategies that I have offered for fibromyalgia and headaches will be useful to those with other illnesses or conditions that interfere with sleep. Just as our physical well-being can affect our sleep, our emotional well-being can affect our sleep, and vice versa. Let's take a look at the complex relationship between emotional well-being and sleep.

* *10* *

Emotional Well-Being and Sleep

Everyone has times in their life when they feel sad, blue, nervous, or worried. Women (and men for that matter) who are experiencing these feelings often say that they are *depressed*. Yet, in this chapter I focus the discussion on depression and anxiety problems that differ from down, nervous, or blue feelings in three specific ways: the depression or anxiety is more intense; it lasts longer; and the difficulties related to it significantly interfere with productive, effective, and satisfying daytime functioning. Most mood and anxiety disorders are more common in women than in men. In this chapter, I define and describe depression and anxiety disorders, as well as the role of sleep in these emotional difficulties, and I also provide some treatment recommendations.

In the section below, I discuss the symptoms of depression, its possible predisposing factors, and treatment options of depression as well as its effects on sleep.

Depression

Depression is a serious, treatable illness that can occur in anyone, man or woman, at any time, and for various reasons regardless of age, race, or income. It affects more than 19 million American adults each year (National Institute of Mental Health 1999). Beginning in adolescence (between the ages of fourteen and eighteen), women are about two times more likely than men to experience mild depressive symptoms or more severe depressive disorders; this gender difference has been found in many different countries (Nolen-Hoeksema 1998). Approximately 12 million women in the United States experience clinical depression each year (National Institute of Mental Health 1999). About one in every eight women can expect to develop clinical depression during her lifetime; depression occurs most frequently in women between the ages of twenty-five and forty-four. Contrary to popular belief, depression is not a "normal part of being a woman," nor is it a "female weakness."

Depression, or *Major Depressive Disorder*, is a type of mood disorder. Another type of mood disorder, also a form of depression, is *Bipolar Disorder* (formerly called manic depression) causes a person to alternate between depression, a sad, lethargic, despondent state, and mania, an overexcited, hyperactive state. A third type of mood disorder is a recurring depression that occurs during winter's dark months (especially in regions where daylight is minimal in winter), referred to as *Seasonal Affective Disorder*. In this chapter I focus first on major depression and later on anxiety disorders.

Although there is a very specific clinical definition for major depression, the illness comes in many forms. The symptoms discussed below can be used as a general guideline. For a more detailed definition of the various types of depression, refer to the *Diagnostic and Statistical Manual of Mental Disorders (DSM-IV)*, which is published by the American Psychiatric Association (1994) and is available in most public libraries.

The key feature of any depression is a change in mood, which is usually experienced as low mood but may be felt as irritability, a lack of pleasure or interest in normally pleasurable activities, or a loss of energy. In major depression, the mood change is usually distinct and severe, lasting for a significant period of time (at least two weeks). As listed below, a variety of symptoms may accompany the mood change. According to the *DSM-IV*, clinical depression includes at least five of the symptoms below, and one of the first two symptoms (depressed mood or diminished interest) must be among the five symptoms present. (For any one of these behaviors to be considered a symptom, it must represent a change from that individual's ordinary behavior.) Low levels of serotonin and other neurotransmitters are associated with depression.

Symptoms of Depression

* Depressed, irritable, unhappy, hopeless mood

* Loss of interest or pleasure in usual activities

* Increased or decreased weight or appetite

* Increased or decreased sleep

* Slowed or agitated movements and activities

* Fatigue and/or loss of energy

* Feelings of worthlessness and/or guilt

* Difficulties in thinking, concentrating, and/or remembering

* Recurring thoughts of death or suicide

Additionally, some individuals experience anxiety and tend to worry more about their physical health. Others may have problems in their relationships (including their marriage), and they may function less effectively at work. Decreased sex drive may be a problem at times. Increased alcohol and substance use often accompanies depression. Episodes of treated or untreated major depression last, on average, two to eight months, but they can last for any length of time. The intensity of symptoms may vary during an episode.

Why Are Some Women More Likely to Experience Depression?

Many physical factors, such as developmental, reproductive, hormonal, and other biological experiences (e.g., childbirth, infertility, and menopause) may contribute to depression in women (National Institute of Mental Health 1999). Social factors also lead to higher rates of clinical depression among women, including stress from work; family responsibilities; the roles and expectations assumed by women; sexual, physical and emotional abuse; and poverty (Nolen-Hoeksema 1998; Unger and Crawford 1992). One friend and colleague told me about her experience, which included sleep problems, anxiety, and depression triggered by stress at work and home:

> As the mother of four children, I am constantly on the go and need all of the energy I can get. I am always busy with family responsibilities, not to mention the responsibilities I carry as a full-time professional. For me, sleep is absolutely crucial. The problem is that the more sleep I need, the harder it is for me to get it. For years, I suffered from intermittent primary and secondary insomnia [primary insomnia is the inability to fall asleep initially, while secondary insomnia is the awakening in the night and the inability to fall back to sleep]. The symptoms began when low-level anxiety and stress from work, motherhood, and a difficult marriage would build up at night and not allow me to rest. Panic symptoms would occasionally surface when I was worrying about my marital problems, which only made my anxiety and inability to sleep worse. Anyone who has lain awake at night trying to fall asleep will understand how

the frustration of not being able to sleep only added to my bouts of insomnia. Fortunately, though, these bouts remained only occasional for a number of years.

Then, a few years ago, I suffered severe depression following the death of my sister. I was clinically depressed and had chronic sleep problems as a result. The insomnia was now constant, always frustrating and always exhausting. I tried many different antidepressants, but most of them left me so exhausted that I felt I was unable to function in daily life. In the end, Ativan (a benzodiazepine) seemed to work best for me, and currently I am sleeping fine with a lower-level antidepressant as well. I have also benefitted from psychotherapy. However, I still have to be careful and I actively avoid anything that might trigger the insomnia again, such as caffeine and work stress.

As I mentioned above, gender differences in depression are remarkably consistent in many cultures—women tend to be more likely than men to become depressed. This consistency suggests that something to do with women's biology may place them at risk for depression. However, numerous studies indicate that this is not the case. For example, women do not seem to have greater deficiencies in neurotransmitters than do men (Blehar and Oren 1995). Many people, including women themselves, believe that women's moods (and thus their depression symptoms) are tied to their hormones. Yet, again, there is little evidence to support such a belief. Studies have not found significant associations between menstrual cycle phase and moods (Parlee 1994) (although a small number of women experience an increase in depressive symptoms during the premenstrual phase [PMS] or in the postpartum period; see chapters 2 and 5). In general, the belief that depression in women is tied to their hormones is not well supported by research. Furthermore, researchers have not found a particular hormone or biochemical abnormality that distinguishes women who experience depression during periods of hormone fluctuation from women who do not experience such depressive episodes. So if the prevalence of depression in women is not due to biological factors, how can it be explained? Below, I examine other possible explanations of the higher incidence of depression among women.

One of the leading experts on the subject of sex differences in depression, Susan Nolen-Hoeksema (1990), compared coping strategies that women and men use to handle stressful situations. She found that when women feel sad or distressed, they are more likely to focus on their distress and passively ruminate about it, while men are more likely to take action to distract themselves or to change the situation. Nolen-Hoeksema (1995) also found that individuals who react with a ruminative response when they are distressed have longer and more severe bouts of depression. This response style may be a contributor to women's higher rates of depression.

Social and cultural forces may also help explain the rates of depression among women. The most compelling social explanation is women's lower socioeconomic status, which puts them at risk for a variety of difficulties, particularly physical and sexual abuse, which often lead to depression. Women are far more likely than men to be the victims of rape, incest, battering, or sexual harassment (Koss, Heise, and Russo 1994). Survivors of physical and sexual assault experience high rates of depression, anxiety disorders, and substance abuse. Undoubtedly, the higher rates of depression in women may be tied to these terrible abuse experiences (Strickland 1992; Laurence and Weinhouse 1994).

Sleep irregularities are often intricately connected with depression and stressful experiences, such as physical or sexual abuse, financial crises, and worries about relationships or work. In the next section, I characterize the sleep changes associated with major depression.

Depression and Sleep Alterations

Disturbed sleep is a characteristic symptom experienced by women and men with depression, and changes in sleep patterns are part of the diagnostic criteria (see "Symptoms of Depression" above). In surveys of the general adult population, 14 to 20 percent of the participants with significant insomnia complaints have shown signs of depression, while only 1 percent of those without sleep complaints displayed signs of depression. In addition, patients with sleep apnea, narcolepsy, or other sleep disorders seem to have higher rates of anxiety, depression, and substance abuse (Benca 2000).

Historically, it has been assumed that depression brings about changes in sleep-wake patterns. However, sleep changes or sleep disorders may affect or contribute to the development of depression. Electroencephalographic (EEG) studies and subjective reports show a tendency toward irregular sleep patterns in depressed adults. Although no single sleep factor reliably distinguishes depressed individuals from those who are not experiencing depression, various changes in sleep patterns, when viewed as a group, provide a picture of how sleep difficulties manifest themselves in depression (Brunello, Armitage, Feinberg, Holsboer-Trachsler, Leger, Linkowski, Mendelson, Racagni, Saletu, Sharpley, Turek, Van Cauter, and Mendlewicz 2000). Sleep changes associated with depression may be grouped into three main categories (Benca 2000):

* Sleep continuity disturbances. Depressed individuals may take longer to fall asleep, experience increased wakefulness during sleep, awaken early in the morning, and have decreased total sleep (Kupfer, Ulrich, and Coble 1985).

* Slow-wave sleep deficits. Many individuals with depression appear to have decreased amounts of slow-wave sleep (Benca 2000).

* Rapid Eye Movement (REM) sleep changes. The period of time from sleep onset to REM onset is significantly reduced in depressed individuals. They also experience prolongation of the first REM period of the night, increased total number of eye movements during the night, and an increased percentage of total REM sleep (Kupfer and Foster 1972).

Researchers disagree about which sleep variables are most problematic for people with depression; however, persistent sleep disturbances are associated with both the relapse and the recurrence of major depression (Ford and Kamerow 1989). In one longitudinal study of young adult men and women, the researchers concluded that nightly insomnia and other sleep disturbances for two weeks or more may be a risk factor for the future onset of major depression (Breslau, Roth, Rosenthal, and Andreski 1996).

The diagnosis of depression in people with sleep problems is often complicated by the fact that many individuals do not recognize the symptoms. Women (and men) may come to their health-care provider or sleep clinic with complaints of insomnia alone. Individuals with depression are sometimes unaware that they are depressed and, instead, attribute their fatigue, poor concentration, and lack of interest to sleep loss. It is also not uncommon for psychologists, social workers, and psychiatrists to diagnose a person with depression when, in fact, the primary difficulty may be insomnia or sleep apnea, with secondary symptoms of depression.

Because depression is often associated with sleep problems and other medical conditions such as alcoholism, eating disorders, and cardiovascular disease, it is important to describe all of your symptoms to your health-care provider, so he or she can conduct a thorough assessment, diagnosis, and treatment of any health problems you may have. A correct diagnosis, whether the main problem is major depression or primary insomnia, will determine the course of treatment. Treatment of sleep complaints associated with depression can have a positive impact for many individuals. Correspondingly, effective treatment of depression can also be a critical aspect of improving sleep. Below are some of the interventions that you may want to consider using for your depression, particularly if you are having sleep problems

Interventions for Depression

Major depression and its accompanying sleep difficulties may be treated with medication, psychotherapy, or a combination of these. If you suspect that you are suffering from depression, it is important that you seek professional help from your health-care provider, who should refer you to a psychiatric social worker, psychiatric nurse, clinical or counseling psychologist, or a psychiatrist. The two most effective psychotherapeutic approaches for depression are cognitive-behavioral therapy and interpersonal therapy, although interpersonal psychotherapy does not tend to focus on the sleep problems associated with depression. Numerous studies have shown that 60 to 70 percent of depressed individuals experience complete relief from their symptoms with twelve weeks of cognitive-behavioral therapy (Futterman, Thompson, Gallagher-Thompson, and Ferris 1995). Cognitive-behavioral approaches to treating depression have two main goals: first, to change patterns of negative, hopeless thinking, and, second, to help depressed women (and men) develop problem-solving skills that in turn allow them to become more effective and more positive in their everyday lives (Lewinsohn, Hoberman, Teri, and Hautziner 1985; Burns 1989). Generally speaking, in this approach a psychotherapist helps a client to challenge negative thoughts, think about possible alternative ways of viewing the situation at hand, and take more effective actions. As discussed in chapter 7, cognitive-behavioral approaches are also often used in treating insomnia. Here are the basic steps used in cognitive-behavioral and social-support approaches to treating depression.

* Keep records of the negative, dysfunctional, automatic thoughts that lead to your negative feelings.

* Challenge your negative thoughts, and determine alternative interpretations or ways of thinking about particularly negative events or situations in your life.

* Work to realize that even if you have to deal with the worst possible situation you can find a beneficial, more positive way of coping with the event(s).

* Plan pleasant events by making and sticking with simple plans, breaking tasks down into small components, and giving yourself credit for whatever you accomplish.

* Build a strong support system. Choose individuals who can empathize with you, affirm your strengths, join you in fun activities, be open-minded about you and your experiences, and accept your ups and downs.

* Finally, work with a professional psychotherapist to learn new coping skills and new ways of handling daily hassles and negative, stressful events.

I recommend that you consult *The Depression Workbook*, by Mary Ellen Copeland and Matthew McKay (1992), and *The Feeling Good Handbook*, by David Burns (1989), for additional self-help advice if you are struggling with depression.

Another highly effective approach to treating depression is interpersonal psychotherapy, in which 60 to 80 percent of depressed individuals recover (Markowitz and Weissman 1995). Interpersonal psychotherapy focuses on a client's interpersonal relationships that may be contributing to her depression. Four main types of interpersonal relationship problems are focused on with this approach to psychotherapy—grief from the loss of a significant relationship (e.g., death of spouse); interpersonal role disputes (e.g., marital difficulties); role transitions (e.g., becoming a mother); and deficits in interpersonal relationship skills (e.g., social isolation).

Studies have demonstrated that cognitive-behavioral, interpersonal, and drug therapies are equally effective in treating most individuals with depression, particularly those who are only moderately depressed (Jacobson and Hollon 1996). Antidepressants are most effective for individuals who are moderately to severely depressed. Yet, often treatment that includes the use of an antidepressant medication works faster than psychotherapy alone.

Therefore, if you are suffering from depression, I encourage you to seek assistance from a psychologist, social worker, or other health-care provider who can provide psychotherapy, in addition to medication if appropriate. Women (and men) who make use of cognitive-behavioral or interpersonal psychotherapies are less likely to relapse with new episodes of depression within two years than those who are on antidepressants alone (Jacobson and Hollon 1996). Furthermore, continuing to see a psychotherapist and to use antidepressant medications for maintenance purposes may reduce the risk of relapse for women (and men) with a history of recurring major depression.

Medical interventions for depression accompanied by sleep difficulties.

If you experience insomnia-like symptoms with your depression, then the approaches used for treating insomnia (discussed in chapter 7) will be beneficial for you. In this section, however, I focus on drug treatments for depression and their effect on sleep. Slightly over one-half of all depressed individuals improve regardless of the type of medication (Benca 2000), but individual women may respond differently to particular drugs. As a result, it is crucial for you to discuss your symptoms and other factors carefully with your healthcare provider when considering an antidepressant medication. For example, individuals with a more agitated depression and severe insomnia might need to be started on a more sedating antidepressant (see the table on the next page for a description of antidepressants, their side effects, and effects on sleep).

The newest class of antidepressant medications, first offered to the public in 1986 with the introduction of Prozac, is the group of selective serotonin reuptake inhibitors (SSRIs). SSRIs are the most widely prescribed drugs for depression in the United States. Along with a few other antidepressants (e.g., bupropion, nefazodone, mirtazapine, and venlafaxine) they have become first-choice medications for depression because of their safety and limited side effects (Benca 2000). However, SSRIs, along with bupropion and venlafaxine, can cause considerable sleep disruption and increase insomnia symptoms for some individuals, whereas nefazodone and mirtazapine are more sedating and may reduce problems with falling asleep and staying asleep.

A second class of antidepressants is the group of tricyclics, which help to reduce the symptoms of depression by changing the levels of norepinephrine, serotonin and other neurotransmitters in the synapse. Although tricyclics are used less frequently because of their side effects, they may be more effective for patients whose symptoms do not improve with the SSRIs or other new antidepressants. Most tricyclics are rather sedating and, as a result, may be helpful for individuals with depression and insomnia symptoms. In fact, low doses of these antidepressants, such as amitriptyline, are commonly prescribed for insomnia (Benca 2000).

A third class of antidepressants is the monoamine oxidase inhibitors (MAOIs) group. MAO is an enzyme that causes the breakdown of the monoamine neurotransmitters, which help prevent symptoms of depression, in the synapse. MAOIs decrease the action of MAO and, therefore, increase the levels of the neurotransmitters in the synapse. Women (and men) whose symptoms do not improve with any of the antidepressants discussed above, and those with atypical symptoms (e.g., hypersomnia, increased appetite, or anxiety), may respond to the MAOIs.

I recommend, as do others in the field, that the choice of antidepressant be closely tied to the individual's dominant sleep problems (Benca 2000). For example, for depression that is associated with insomnia symptoms, the more sedating antidepressants, tricyclics such as Elavil and Pamelor (see table), are most beneficial and should be administered in a single dose at bedtime (Benca 2000). On the other hand, sometimes insomnia occurs as a side effect of SSRIs and, as a

Medications for Depression and Their Side Effects

Medication	Side Effects	Sleep Effects
Selective serotonin reuptake inhibitors (SSRIs): fluoxetine (Prozac), paroxetine (Paxil), sertraline (Zoloft), trazodone (Desyrel), nefazodone (Serzone)	Stomach disturbances, sexual dysfunction, anxiety, agitation, dizziness, dry mouth	Insomnia, REM suppression, increased slow-wave sleep, sedation
Tricyclics: amitriptyline (Elavil), imipramine (Tofranil), doxepin (Sinequan), nortriptyline (Pamelor), desipramine (Norpramin)	Blurred vision, dry mouth, urinary retention, flushing, rapid heartbeat, liver toxicity, weight gain	Sedation, REM sleep suppression, increased Stage 2 sleep
Monoamine oxidase inhibitors (MAOIs)	Hypertensive crisis with tyramine-containing foods, dizziness, agitation, liver toxicity, weight gain	Insomnia, REM sleep suppression
Bupropion (Wellbutrin)	Stomach upset, lowered seizure threshold	Insomnia, increased REM sleep
Venlafaxine (Effexor)	Anxiety, anorexia	Insomnia
Mirtazapine (Remeron)	Increased appetite, weight gain, dizziness	Sedation

(adapted from Benca 2000)

result, requires additional medications. If insomnia becomes a problem while you are taking SSRIs, consult your health-care provider. He or she may consider adjusting your current medication or giving you an additional medication to improve your sleep. Behavioral therapies (discussed in chapter 7) may also be helpful for individuals with depression and coexisting insomnia. Of course, good sleep habits are beneficial to everyone, particularly those with depression and insomnia. Caffeine, nicotine, and alcohol use are discouraged for individuals suffering from insomnia. Finally, studies have shown that bright-light therapy, either alone or in combination with antidepressant medications, may be beneficial to those with winter depression and excessive daytime sleepiness (see chapter 7 for a description of light therapy).

Sleep deprivation as a method for treating depression.

Sleep clinicians and researchers are beginning to consider sleep- schedule changes as a treatment alternative for depression, since it appears that some individuals experience improved or elevated mood following a single night of sleep deprivation. Approaches include selective deprivation of REM sleep, partial and total sleep deprivation, and phase advance of sleep (in which bedtime is gradually moved to an earlier time). However, such sleep countermeasures are not being widely used and should not be tried without professional advice. Studies suggest that severely depressed women and men may benefit more from sleep deprivation than those who are mildly depressed, but that healthy, nondepressed individuals actually experience increased depressed mood following such sleep deprivation (Pilcher and Huffcutt 1996). Unfortunately, however, the positive effects of sleep deprivation as a therapeutic technique for depression are short lived, since depression symptoms return immediately after the person sleeps, even in a short nap.

Many antidepressants have REM-suppressant effects. In fact, researchers have theorized that certain antidepressants, including MAOIs, tricyclics, and SSRIs, may be effective because of selective REM sleep deprivation. However, since some of the newer antidepressants do not suppress REM sleep, it is possible that REM suppression may not be necessary for reducing depression symptoms.

When you meet with your health-care provider to discuss your concerns regarding depression, carefully describe your sleep difficulties, since such symptoms may influence the course of treatment: for individuals with excessive daytime sleepiness, antidepressants that cause alertness may be most effective, while depressed women with insomnia are likely to do better with a sedating antidepressant. in both cases, it is recommended that medication be combined with cognitive behavioral therapy.

Like people with depression, individuals with anxiety problems often have coexisting sleep problems. Below is a discussion of some of the primary anxiety disorders, their sleep features, and some treatment recommendations.

Anxiety

As most of us realize, anxiety is an inevitable part of life. In fact, at this very moment I am quite anxious about finishing this book in time for its planned publication date; as a result, I am not sleeping well and feel tense and uneasy. Years ago, as a college and graduate student, I often felt anxious during exams, and in my early years of teaching, I often felt anxious when speaking in front of my classes. Many people feel anxious when peering down from a high ledge, traveling in an airplane, or while waiting to play in a basketball game. Most people probably feel some anxiety at some point during their life. Fortunately for most of us, the uneasiness is not intense and persistent, and it does not interfere with our everyday responsibilities. On the other hand, if your anxiety is ongoing and debilitating, you may have an anxiety disorder, marked by distressing, persistent anxiety and fear that often interfere with daily functioning (American Psychiatric Association 1994). Four different types of symptoms make up what clinicians refer to as an anxiety disorder (Nolen-Hoeksema 1998). First, somatic symptoms include dizziness, sweating palms, heart palpitations, dry mouth and throat, and periods of shaking. Second, emotional symptoms include fearfulness and vigilance against impending panic attacks. Third, cognitive symptoms include unrealistic worries about negative events. Fourth, behavioral symptoms include avoidance of certain situations that are frightening to the sufferer.

Below are definitions of the four most common anxiety disorders:

* Panic Disorder. In this disorder, the sufferer experiences sudden episodes of intense dread in which he or she feels terror and accompanying heart palpitations, choking, dizziness, shortness of breath, and/or other frightening sensations.

* Generalized Anxiety Disorder. The person has unexplained and continuous feelings of uneasiness and anxiety.

* Phobias. These are irrational fears of a specific object or situation (e.g., heights, closed-in spaces, flying, or crossing bridges), and avoidance of that object or situation.

* Obsessive-Compulsive Disorder. This condition is characterized by unwanted repetitive thoughts and/or actions, and is sometimes

accompanied by difficulty falling asleep and decreased total sleep time.

In the remaining part of this chapter, I focus mainly on Panic Disorder and Generalized Anxiety Disorder, because they illustrate the sleep problems that can coexist with any of the anxiety disorders, particularly phobias, and because research to date has focused on these two disorders. Different anxiety disorders appear to be associated with different types and severities of sleep disturbances. Individuals with phobias have minimal sleep difficulties except for those whose phobia is linked with their sleeping environment, while some individuals with Obsessive-Compulsive Disorder have poor-quality sleep (Uhde 2000). Let's now take a look at the relationship between sleep and panic disorder.

Panic Disorder and Sleep

Between 8 and 12 percent of individuals have occasional panic attacks, especially during periods of intense stress (Telch, Lucas, and Nelson 1989). Yet, when panic attacks become frequent, spontaneous, and worrisome, and the person changes behavior in attempt to avoid such attacks, then a diagnosis of Panic Disorder may be given. Panic Disorder affects nearly two to three times more women than men, and the average age for initial panic attacks is twenty-two years, although even children can experience panic attacks.

The symptoms of a panic attack include: pounding heartbeat; numbness or tingling sensations in the hands or feet; chills or hot flashes; sweating; trembling; shortness of breath; feeling of choking or chest discomfort; nausea and upset stomach; dizziness, light-headedness, or faintness; feelings of being detached from oneself; fear of losing control; and fear of dying (American Psychiatric Association 1994). If you experience intense fear or discomfort and develop at least four of these symptoms, which start abruptly and peak within ten minutes, you are probably having a panic attack. When panic attacks occur frequently and interfere with daily living, you may have Panic Disorder. The frequency and pattern of panic attacks varies from one person to the next. Some women (and men) have attacks every day for a week and then go for weeks or months without having another attack. Others have attacks less often but more regularly, such as once a week for several months.

The official diagnosis of panic attacks and disorder does not include sleep panic attacks (Uhde 2000). However, more clinicians and researchers are recognizing that panic attacks can occur during sleep, particularly late in Stage 2 or early Stage 3 sleep (Uhde 2000). This experience is referred to as *sleep panic* or *nocturnal panic*. For those who experience sleep panic, it can be a terribly scary and disruptive experience. One friend shared her rather trying experience:

> I've had these panic attacks during the night for at least ten years. I am suddenly awakened from sleep without any recollection of having been asleep or dreaming. When I have these attacks, I awaken with a sense of doom and dread, intense heart palpitations, shortness of breath, and sometimes nausea. These symptoms usually last for several minutes. Often I feel so scared that I wake up my husband as well. I tend to experience more of these sleep attacks when I am under pressure at work, such as when I'm working to meet a paper deadline, or doing a lot of traveling. After a night with one or two attacks, I often have trouble falling back to sleep, have difficulty getting up in the morning, and, as a result, feel exhausted the following day. I rarely have panic attacks during the day and in fact it took me a while to seek help since I had never heard of having panic attacks at night.
>
> I am now doing far better. I was on a low dose of imipramine, and now I am working with a psychologist to learn how to handle my anxiety symptoms and irrational thoughts that I have regarding stressful situations.

Insomnia, restless, or erratic sleep and nocturnal panic attacks are common symptoms for individuals with panic disorder (Mellman and Uhde 1989). Approximately 65 percent of individuals with Panic Disorder have a history of nighttime panic attacks, and it is not uncommon for those with Panic Disorder to say that their sleep panic attacks are the most disturbing and disruptive aspect of the disorder. Sleep panic symptoms are similar in quality, severity, and duration to daytime panic attacks. As you would expect, individuals with Panic Disorder and nocturnal attacks report far more insomnia symptoms, particularly frequent awakenings throughout the night, than do those who don't have sleep panic attacks (Hauri, Friedman, and Ravaris 1989).

The most worrisome complication of nocturnal panic is chronic, intermittent sleep deprivation (Craske and Barlow 1989). As nocturnal panic attacks worsen, individuals begin to fear going to sleep. As a result, they avoid going to bed and become increasingly more sleep deprived, and their anxiety symptoms escalate. Individuals with sleep panic are often embarrassed about their fear and avoidance of sleep, and so they may create excuses for their poor sleep habits, telling themselves things like, "I have too much work to do to go to bed." They may instead attempt to get rest without actually falling asleep. If you experience sleep panic, you may find yourself trying any of the following tactics: sitting up in bed, sitting in a armchair and watching a late-night movie, lying down in bed without getting under the covers, or asking your partner to watch you sleep so that they are available if you have a nocturnal panic attack. In fact, individuals who experience sleep panic often feel relieved to be evaluated in a sleep clinic because they know they will be watched while they are sleeping.

So, if you struggle with chronic daytime or nighttime panic attacks, what are your treatment options? As is the case with depression and other mood disorders, several strategies, discussed below, are effective in the treatment of Panic Disorder. Consult your health-care provider to find out what strategies might be right for you.

Understanding and Treating Panic Disorder

What causes Panic Disorder? Certain people seem to have a biological or psychological predisposition for the development of this anxiety disorder. When they experience just a mild stimulus, some individuals respond with fear, a pounding heartbeat, rapid breathing, sweaty palms, and other symptoms. When these people overfocus on such bodily sensations, they may interpret the sensations in a negative manner (e.g., believing they are having a heart attack or going crazy) and engage in snowballing, catastrophic thinking, which leads to a panic attack (Barlow 1988). Put another way, this kind of thinking actually increases the intensity of their initially mild physiological symptoms to the level of a panic attack. Often, following an initial panic attack, individuals become hypervigilant, always looking out for signs and signals of the start of another attack. Unfortunately, this constant anxiety increases the likelihood that additional panic attacks will happen.

As with the treatment of depression, drug therapy and psychotherapy are both useful in the treatment of Panic Disorder. The aim of both forms of treatment is to block panic attacks and eliminate secondary fears and avoidance behaviors.

Surprisingly, some of the most effective medications for the treatment of Panic Disorder are antidepressants. For example, tricyclic antidepressants, such as imipramine and amitriptyline, can reduce panic attacks in 60 to 90 percent of individuals, particularly typical daytime panic attacks (Lydiard, Brawman-Mintzer, and Ballenger 1996). SSRIs, such as fluoxetine, commonly known as Prozac, are also effective in reducing panic attacks (Uhde 2000). However, if your health-care provider prescribes Prozac, it will be important for you to watch for insomnia, a common side effect of Prozac, since lack of sleep can make your Panic Disorder worse. Other side effects are listed in the table entitled "Medications for Depression and Their Side Effects" earlier in the chapter.

High-potency benzodiazepines, such as alprazolam (Xanax), are also used to treat Panic Disorder. These medications quickly reduce panic attacks, particularly their intensity, and other general anxiety symptoms in 60 to 80 percent of individuals with Panic Disorder (Klosko, Barlow, Tassinari, and Ceerny 1990). Unfortunately, Xanax and other benzodiazepines have several significant disadvantages. First, they are physically and psychologically addictive. Women (and men) build up a tolerance so that they need increasing dosages of the medication to get a positive effect. Second, benzodiazepines can interfere with a person's ability to function and perform activities like driving a car. Third, most individuals relapse after being taken off these medications (Fryer, Liebowitz, Gorman, and Campeas 1987). Finally, when a person stops taking Xanax or other similar medication, she is likely to experience some of the following symptoms: irritability, tremors, insomnia, tingling sensations, and, more rarely, paranoid thoughts.

Far less information regarding the treatment of sleep panic attacks is available. A small number of studies have found that tricyclic antidepressants are effective in reducing nocturnal panic attacks in individuals with a history of both daytime and nighttime panic attacks (Uhde 2000). Individuals who experience sleep panic attacks as well as sleep deprivation are often treated with tricyclics and encouraged to develop good sleep habits.

Moreover, cognitive-behavioral techniques such as relaxation exercises and psychotherapy are also valuable in reducing day and nighttime panic attacks and the accompanying avoidance behaviors, especially when learned and practiced with the help of a health-care provider. There are four basic components of a cognitive-behavioral approach to treating Panic Disorder:

1. Learn progressive relaxation (see appendix B) and breathing exercises. Relaxation will help you gain control over your anxiety symptoms; eventually you will find that you are able to use your relaxation techniques as a counterresponse to your anxiety symptoms (e.g., rapid breathing, heart palpitations, sweaty palms, and so on).

2. Identify the thoughts that reinforce and perpetuate the body sensations that accompany your panic attacks. Try keeping a panic-thoughts diary or chart. In keeping a chart you may notice that you tend to have panic symptoms during the night or while in your office at work. You might note in your diary, for instance, that you felt moderate to severe dizziness, had a racing heartbeat, and experienced some sweating in these situations. You might also keep track of what you were thinking just before a panic attack started. Once you learn what situations and thoughts tend

to bring on your panic symptoms, you'll more readily be able to call upon your new relaxation techniques to block panic attacks.

3. Use the relaxation and breathing exercises while you are experiencing panic symptoms. (You may want to practice the skills while you are in session with your psychotherapist.) After a while, you will find that you are using the relaxation techniques automatically, preventing a full-blown attack.

4. Learn new ways of thinking about and interpreting the body sensations that accompany panic. For example, if you tend to interpret your heart palpitations as the start of a heart attack, your anxiety naturally increases and further exacerbates your panic symptoms; to reverse this thought process, your therapist can help you gather evidence from your doctor or nurse practitioner that shows you have excellent cardiac health and are unlikely to have a heart attack. Then you can learn to remind yourself, whenever you feel a panic attack starting. that you are not having a heart attack. By learning to interpret your body's sensations in a more positive, constructive manner, you will decrease your anxiety level and diminish the likelihood of additional panic attacks. If you tend to experience sleep panic attacks and you fear going to sleep, try reminding yourself that you are not going to die if you go to sleep; try to think of sleep instead as something positive and nourishing for you body. This will make it easier for you to begin to return to healthy sleep behaviors (such as sleeping in bed instead of in a chair in the family room) and eventually uninterrupted nighttime sleep.

Whether you use drug therapy, psychotherapy, or both, you will need to also eliminate habits or behaviors that make your Panic Disorder worse, such as allowing yourself to become sleep deprived, or using caffeine. You'll also need to take care of yourself and practice doing things that make you feel good.

Generalized Anxiety Disorder and Sleep Complaints

Another anxiety difficulty that includes sleep problems is referred to as Generalized Anxiety Disorder (GAD). The hallmark of this particular anxiety disorder is unrelenting anxiety in almost all situations. If one of your friends had Generalized Anxiety Disorder, you would probably describe her as nervous, tense, uptight, and always worrying. People with GAD experience muscle tension, sleep disturbances, and chronic restlessness. GAD symptoms affect women and men equally (Uhde 2000).

Over half of the individuals with GAD have trouble sleeping (Hoehn-Sarc and McLeod 1990). Similar to those who experience insomnia, some women with GAD say that during the day they cannot stop worrying or thinking about the problems they will have at bedtime when they try to sleep. Usually, individuals with GAD say that they have difficulties falling asleep and staying asleep, experiencing restless, fragmented sleep throughout the night (Uhde 2000).

Treatment options for Generalized Anxiety Disorder.

Benzodiazepines have traditionally been the main treatment for GAD. Although this is still the case, SSRIs are also useful in treating this disorder. Since many individuals with GAD also experience insomnia, any treatment program should focus on reducing the insomnia in addition to the other anxiety symptoms. See chapter 7 for a detailed discussion of cognitive-behavioral treatment for insomnia.

*   *   *   *   *

Depression and anxiety disorders are often, but not always, associated with difficulty falling and staying asleep, as well as excessive daytime sleepiness. The role of sleep deprivation in mood and anxiety disorders is not entirely understood and requires further research. Recent research indicates that anxiety disorders can be distinguished from major depression with regard to sleep deprivation: individuals with depression tend to experience at least temporary improvement following sleep deprivation, whereas those who struggle with anxiety disorders report that their symptoms either worsen (in the case of Panic Disorder) or do not change (in the case of Generalized Anxiety Disorder) after sleep loss. If you are struggling with an anxiety or mood disorder together with sleep difficulties, it is crucial that you make sure that your health-care provider recognizes your sleep disturbances and focuses treatment in a way that lessens both your symptoms of depression or anxiety as well as your sleep disturbances. Effective treatment of the core symptoms of most mood and anxiety disorders will almost always result in a corresponding improvement in sleep problems. If sleep disturbances continue after your mood disorder symptoms get better, you and your health-care provider should reassess your symptoms for other possible medical or sleep disorders. In some situations it may be appropriate to focus on the sleep problems as a separate, primary issue as opposed to treating them as a secondary, less significant concern.

* *

Conclusion

As you now know, sleep-wake patterns change throughout women's lives due to changes in responsibilities and circumstances, and as a result of changes in our hormone levels during the month and as we age. Some women do not notice these changes and may even think of themselves as great sleepers, while others have difficulty with sleep at some point in their life.

In my opinion, women's health and, specifically, women's sleep must become a priority in research, in clinical practice, and in women's own lives. Women's health issues, and now sleep issues, are at the forefront of our cultural consciousness as never before. I believe that in order to have some control over our lives and be informed participants in our health care, we need knowledge about our bodies. As the authors of *Our Bodies, Ourselves* (Boston Women's Health Book Collective 1998) emphasize, knowledge gives us the ability to make informed choices and decisions, and it gives us some of the control that we all want and need. Today there is far more health and medical information available than there was two decades ago. However, it is crucial that we obtain information from sources that are timely, accurate, user friendly, and beneficial to women. It is my hope that this book on women's sleep fits that description, and that it will become a part of your library on women's health.

As a result of reading this book, you may now be more savvy regarding the relationship between sleep and health than some health-care professionals, so do not be afraid to voice your opinions and your needs when you're seeking health care. Consumers and health-care providers must collaborate as we gain new knowledge regarding sleep, circadian rhythms, sleep disorders, and related overall health.

Finally, I hope you realize after reading and sleeping on this book that women's sleep-wake habits are influenced by a variety of factors—age, hormones, life stage, stress levels, mood, parental status, work hours, and so on. Moreover, the quality, quantity, and nature of sleep affect women's emotional and physical well-being. Unquestionably, women need to take an active role in examining their sleep habits as they relate to work and family responsibilities, mood fluctuations, and other aspects of daytime functioning and self-care.

Although sleep needs vary from woman to woman, the majority of women (and men) require approximately 7.5 to 8 hours of sleep to cope with work duties, family demands, driving, and other responsibilities. When women do not get enough sleep, their physical and emotional health is put at risk. I hope that after reading this book you are more knowledgeable about women's sleep and your own sleep needs, and that you feel prepared to try to improve your sleep and your overall health. I wish you restful sleep and sweet dreams.

Appendix A

Glossary of Terms

Analgesic: Medication or treatment that is used to relieve pain.

Apneic event: Involuntary pause in breathing.

Arthritis: Joint inflammation; affects the joints and other connective tissues of the body, including muscles, tendons, and ligaments, as well as the protective covering of internal organs.

Autoimmune disease: Disease in which the immune system destroys or attacks one's own body tissue.

Central sleep apnea: Sleep disorder in which the brain fails to send signals to respiration muscles, resulting in restricted breathing.

Chronic insomnia: Inadequate or poor-quality sleep occurring on most nights and lasting a month or more.

Circadian rhythm: A cyclical rhythm that lasts for approximately twenty-four hours. Circadian rhythms regulate sleep, activity, body temperature, hormone secretion, and a number of other physiological variables. Often called a "biological rhythm."

Collagen: Structural protein of the skin, tendons, bone cartilage, and connective tissues.

Continuous Positive Airway-Pressure Treatment (CPAP): The most common treatment used in sleep apnea patients. Continuous airway pressure is supplied through the patient's nasal passages by a special mask worn over the nose during sleep.

Corpus luteum: The follicle from which an ovum has burst. As the corpus luteum recovers from being burst, it produces estrogen and, in larger amounts, progesterone, the necessary hormone for maintenance of a pregnancy.

Dopamine agonist: A medication that serves as a substitute for dopamine.

Dysmenorrhea: Commonly known as menstrual cramps, dysmenorrhea includes spasmodic cramping and congestive cramping (which causes the body to retain fluids and salts).

EEG (electroencephalogram): Measurement of brain waves using an electroencephalograph; can be seen when there is a change in voltage between two bits of metal, called "electrodes," attached to the scalp. EEG voltage changes are measured as changes in duration (cycles per second) and amplitude (microvolts).

EMG (electromyogram): Measurement of muscle activity using an electromyograph; voltage changes are detected through electrodes placed on the surface of skin overlying muscles. Muscles under the chin show the most dramatic changes in muscle activity associated with various sleep stages.

Endometrium: The surface of the uterine lining; becomes increasingly covered with mucus during menstruation.

EOG (electrooculogram): Measurement of eye movements; when an electrode is placed on the skin near the eye, it records a change in voltage as the eye rotates in its socket.

Esophageal reflux: Commonly referred to as heartburn, this disorder occurs when the lower esophageal sphincter is loose and allows stomach acids to enter the esophagus.

Estrogen: A sex hormone, made by the maturing follicle, that causes the uterine lining (endometrium) to grow, thicken, form glands, and increase uterine blood supply. Levels of estrogen peak during ovulation.

Ferritin: A body chemical that indicates stores of iron.

Fetal Alcohol Syndrome: Group of fetal abnormalities caused by a mother's consumption of alcohol during pregnancy. Abnormalities include problems such as growth retardation, defects in facial features, and intellectual retardation.

Fibromyalgia: Disorder that causes chronic pain and stiffness throughout the tissues that support and move bones and joints.

Fibrous capsule: The tendons and ligaments that wrap around joints.

FSH-RF: A chemical released by the hypothalamus, it activates the pituitary gland during menstruation. The pituitary gland is responsible for secreting hormones that cause a follicle to mature.

Hormone replacement therapy (HRT): Drug treatment that combines estrogen and progestin (a form of progesterone) to keep hormone levels sustained within a normal range during menopause. Along with reducing hot flashes and nighttime sweats, hormone replacement therapy reduces the risk of osteoporosis and may prevent heart disease.

Hot flashes: Sudden increases in heart rate and peripheral blood flow that cause a rise in skin temperature and, as a result, sweating.

Following a hot flash, sweat evaporates and the body cools down, resulting in a chilled feeling.

Hypothalamus: A neural structure lying below the thalamus, in the brain. It directs several activities that are related to maintenance of the body, such as eating, drinking, body temperature, and menstruation, and it helps govern the endocrine system through the pituitary gland.

Indeterminant sleep: Poorly organized sleep of infants; a state of sleep that can neither be defined as NREM or REM.

Intermittent insomnia: Inadequate or poor-quality sleep, occurring from time to time.

Insomnia: Inadequate or abnormal sleep. Characteristics include difficulty falling asleep, frequent awakenings during the night, a short sleep time, and generally nonrestorative sleep.

Joint space: Volume that is enclosed within the fibrous capsule and synovium.

k-complexes: These brain waves occur spontaneously during Stage 2 of NREM sleep and may be measured by electrodes on an EEG; they are often accompanied by sleep spindles. They are illustrated by a sharp negative EEG wave followed by a slow wave with high voltage. One way to induce a k-complex is to clap loudly or bang on a door near a sleeping person.

Leutenizing Hormone: A hormone secreted by the pituitary gland and sent into the bloodstream to begin the maturation process of the follicles. As menstruation advances, the pituitary gland releases a larger amount of leutenizing hormone, which eventually triggers one of the most mature follicles to burst open and release an egg.

Lower esophageal sphincter: The valve located between the esophagus and the stomach that allows food and water to pass into the stomach and prevents backward flow of such substances.

Menopause: The conclusion of menstruation; the change is confirmed when no menstrual period has occurred for twelve consecutive months. Menopause marks the end of fertility, resulting from the ovaries' decreased production of the sex hormones estrogen and progesterone.

Multiple Sleep Latency Test (MSLT): Measurement of speed at which an individual falls asleep, the degree of excessive daytime sleepiness, and the likelihood of sleep apnea. For example, if the time it takes to fall asleep is less than five minutes, a sleep disorder such as sleep apnea is likely to be a factor.

Night sweats: Nighttime hot flashes that are particularly severe, resulting in excessive perspiration and increased sleep difficulties.

Non–Rapid Eye Movement (NREM) Sleep: Period of sleep with no visible eye movements or twitches. EEG patterns are synchronized and relatively slow, and the autonomic nervous system functions at a regular pace.

Nonsteroidal anti-inflammatory drugs (NSAIDs): Drugs that are used to reduce inflammation that causes joint pain, stiffness, and swelling (e.g., aspirin).

Obstructive sleep apnea: An event during sleep in which there is no air-flow into the lungs despite the efforts of the respiratory system.

Obstructive Sleep Apnea Syndrome: Sleep disorder characterized by repeated collapse of the upper airway during sleep, leading to decreased airflow, cessation of airflow (apnea) and, ultimately, oxygen desaturation of the hemoglobin. Repeated desaturation can significantly alter normal cardiovascular and pulmonary function, which results in pulmonary and systemic hypertension and cardiac arrhythmias.

Ovulation: The process in which a surge of Leutenizing Hormone causes a follicle to burst and release an egg into the fallopian tube. The egg is then carried toward the uterus, where fertilization may occur.

Periodic Limb Movements: Occurring during sleep, and sometimes during wakefulness, involuntary periodic movements of the legs and/or upper limbs.

Perimenopause: The menopause transition period spanning from four to eight years prior to menopause to the year after menopause.

Phase advance: Shift of the sleep period to an earlier point in the 24-hour continuum (e.g., shift from 11:00 P.M.–7:00 A.M. to 8:00 P.M.– 4:00 A.M. represents a 3-hour phase advance).

Phase delay: Shift of the sleep period to a later point in the 24-hour continuum; the opposite of a phase advance (e.g., shift from 8:00 P.M. –4:00 A.M. to 11:00 P.M.–7:00 A.M. represents a 3-hour phase delay).

Pituitary gland: Located at the base of the brain, it secretes Follicle Stimulating Hormone (FSH) and Leutenizing Hormone (LH) into the bloodstream. Responsible for starting the maturation process of the follicles.

Polysomnographic measures: Simultaneous assessments of different physiological processes during sleep (e.g., eye, muscle, heart, and brain activity).

Polysomnography: A mechanical test used during sleep to record numerous variables including electric activity in the brain, eye movements, muscle activity, heart rate, respiratory effort, air flow, and blood oxygen levels.

Postpartum depression: Depression that occurs in a woman shortly after childbirth.

Postpartum period: The first six months after childbirth.

Postpartum psychosis: A relatively rare disorder that occurs in a woman shortly after childbirth, with symptoms similar to general psychosis, such as confusion, fatigue, agitation, mood swings, feelings of hopelessness and shame, delusions or auditory hallucinations, hyperactivity, and rapid speech or mania.

Preeclampsia: A condition that occurs during pregnancy and includes high blood pressure, sudden weight gain, and other symptoms. Onset is usually after 20 weeks of gestation.

Progestrone: Sex hormone that is necessary for the maintenance of a pregnancy and causes the endometrium to become covered with mucus in preparation for a fertilized egg.

Prostaglandins: The body chemicals that affect muscle tension; they cause spasmodic cramping often associated with the menstrual cycle.

Rapid Eye Movement (REM) Sleep: The sleep state during which rapid eye movements are seen, muscle tone is absent, and the autonomic nervous system shows irregular and accelerated activity.

REM sleep latency: Interval from the time of sleep onset to the first appearance of REM sleep.

Raynaud's Syndrome: The circulatory condition associated with spasms in blood vessels of fingers and toes that cause extremities to change color. When exposed to cold, fingers and toes will turn white, then blue, and then red.

Reconditioning: Treatment for insomnia that helps a patient to reassociate her bed and bedtime with sleep. This requires a patient to use her beds for only sleep and sexual activity.

Relaxation therapy: Treatment for insomnia that uses techniques that reduce or eliminate anxiety and body tension. As a result, a person's mind stops "racing," the muscles relax, and restful sleep can occur.

Restless Legs Syndrome: A motor disorder that is characterized by uncomfortable sensations in the legs. Sensations are described by sufferers as pulling, drawing, crawling, tingling, prickly, and often painful. Usually, the symptoms are accompanied by an overwhelming urge to constantly move the legs.

Sleep apnea: Condition in which an individual stops breathing repeatedly during their sleep. The frequency and time duration of stoppages vary, but the stoppages can occur hundreds of times each night and each last up to a minute or longer. The individual may partially awaken each time an apnea happens, which interferes with restful, continuous sleep. The condition can cause morning headaches, impotence, insomnia, or hypersomnia.

Sleep efficiency: Ratio of one's total sleep time to total time in bed.

Sleep hygiene: To get effective and beneficial sleep, certain conditions and practices that should be maintained. These include a regular bedtime and rise time; restriction of beverages, certain foods, drinks, and drugs before bedtime; and the use of exercise, nutrition, and certain environmental factors to enhance, not disturb, restful sleep.

Sleep latency: Duration of time from bedtime ("lights out") to the onset of sleep. In a laboratory setting, onset of sleep is generally defined as the appearance of three consecutive epochs of Stage 1 sleep or one epoch of any other sleep stage.

Sleep restriction: Treatment program that initially allows only a few hours of sleep during the night. The allowed time is gradually increased until a more normal night's sleep is achieved.

Sleep spindles: A brain-wave formation often seen on an EEG during Stage 2 of NREM sleep; it is recognized by its repeated oscillations at a high frequency, ranging from twelve to fourteen cycles per second.

Sleep stages: The various subdivisions of sleep (wakefulness, Stages 1 through 4, NREM, and REM sleep).

Slow-wave sleep (SWS): Stage 3 of NREM sleep; it is characterized by high-amplitude, slow waves, called "delta waves" that appear on an EEG. Eye movements are rarely seen, and muscle activity is low to moderate.

Stimulants: Drugs (e.g., caffeine, nicotine, and the more powerful amphetamines and cocaine) that excite neural activity and speed up body functions. They interfere with sleep.

Somnoplasty: Procedure used to reduce the size of some airway structures (e.g., uvula or back of the tongue) by applying radio waves to those tissues. The procedure is currently being researched as a treatment for sleep apnea.

Suprachiasmatic nucleus: A group of nerve cells that are located above the optic chiasm; this bundle of cells generates circadian signals for the control of sleep and wakefulness.

Synapse: The site at which a nerve impulse passes from one neuron to another; the junction between the axon tip of the sending neuron and the dendrite or cell body of the receiving neuron.

Synovium: Tissue that surrounds and protects the joints. It produces synovial fluid and it nourishes and lubricates the joints.

Transient insomnia: Inadequate or poor-quality sleep that lasts from a single night to a few weeks.

Uvulopalatopharyngoplasty (UPPP): A surgical procedure that removes excess tissue from the back of the throat (e.g., the tonsils or uvula). Removal of these tissues reduces or eliminates snoring but does not necessarily eliminate sleep apnea.

Uvula: The fleshy mass of tissue that hangs at the center of the back of the throat.

Vasculitis: Inflammation of blood vessels.

Zeitgeber: A time cue in the environment. For example, light, noise, food, social interactions, and an alarm clock can help to keep an individual on a steady schedule throughout a twenty-four-hour day.

* *

Appendix B

Part I: Sleep/Wake Diary

Copy the diary templates on the following pages into a notebook. Keep the diary for at least one week, or longer if you like. Before you go to bed at night, answer the questions on the sheet labeled "Evening Diary." After you have awakened in the morning, answer the morning questions that are on the opposite side of the evening page, labeled "Morning Diary." If a question does not apply to you, do not answer it. Leave that question blank and move on to the next question.

EVENING DIARY

Day/Date	How sleepy did I feel today?	Did I doze off today without planning to? If yes, where?	Did I nap today? If yes, how long, and when?	How much caffeine (e.g., soda, coffee, tea, chocolate) did I have today?	When did I exercise today?	Medications I took during the day	What time did I shower, take a bath, or nap? (Write start time/finish time for each.)
Day 1	1 = extremely 2 = sort of sleepy 3 = not at all	___ Yes ___ No Where? ___	___ Yes ___ No Nap 1: Length ___ Nap 2: Length ___ min. Where? Nap 3: Length ___ min. Where?	Had no caffeine ___ Type and amount ___ Time of day ___ Type and amount ___ Time of day ___ Type and amount ___ Time of day ___	___ No Exercise ___ Morning ___ Afternoon ___ Evening ___ 2–3 hrs before bed	Names of medications	Shower/Bath ___ ___ A.M./P.M. Nap (accidentally fell asleep ___ ___ A.M./P.M.
Day 2	1 = extremely 2 = sort of sleepy 3 = not at all	___ Yes ___ No Where? ___	___ Yes ___ No Nap 1: Length ___ Nap 2: Length ___ min. Where? Nap 3: Length ___ min. Where?	Had no caffeine ___ Type and amount ___ Time of day ___ Type and amount ___ Time of day ___ Type and amount ___ Time of day ___	___ No Exercise ___ Morning ___ Afternoon ___ Evening ___ 2–3 hrs before bed	Names of medications	Shower/Bath ___ ___ A.M./P.M. Nap (accidentally fell asleep ___ ___ A.M./P.M.
Day 3	1 = extremely 2 = sort of sleepy 3 = not at all	___ Yes ___ No Where? ___	___ Yes ___ No Nap 1: Length ___ Nap 2: Length ___ min. Where? Nap 3: Length ___ min. Where?	Had no caffeine ___ Type and amount ___ Time of day ___ Type and amount ___ Time of day ___ Type and amount ___ Time of day ___	___ No Exercise ___ Morning ___ Afternoon ___ Evening ___ 2–3 hrs before bed	Names of medications	Shower/Bath ___ ___ A.M./P.M. Nap (accidentally fell asleep ___ ___ A.M./P.M.

Day 4	1 = extremely 2 = sort of sleepy 3 = not at all	___ Yes ___ No Where?	___ Yes ___ No Nap 1: Length ___ min. Where? Nap 2: Length ___ min. Where? Nap 3: Length ___ min. Where?	Had no caffeine ___ Type and amount ___ Time of day ___ Type and amount ___ Time of day ___ Type and amount ___ Time of day ___	No Exercise ___ Morning ___ Afternoon ___ Evening ___ 2–3 hrs before bed	Names of medications	Shower/Bath ___ A.M./P.M. Nap (accidentally fell asleep) ___ A.M./P.M.
Day 5	1 = extremely 2 = sort of sleepy 3 = not at all	___ Yes ___ No Where?	___ Yes ___ No Nap 1: Length ___ min. Where? Nap 2: Length ___ min. Where? Nap 3: Length ___ min. Where?	Had no caffeine ___ Type and amount ___ Time of day ___ Type and amount ___ Time of day ___ Type and amount ___ Time of day ___	No Exercise ___ Morning ___ Afternoon ___ Evening ___ 2–3 hrs before bed	Names of medications	Shower/Bath ___ A.M./P.M. Nap (accidentally fell asleep) ___ A.M./P.M.
Day 6	1 = extremely 2 = sort of sleepy 3 = not at all	___ Yes ___ No Where?	___ Yes ___ No Nap 1: Length ___ min. Where? Nap 2: Length ___ min. Where? Nap 3: Length ___ min. Where?	Had no caffeine ___ Type and amount ___ Time of day ___ Type and amount ___ Time of day ___ Type and amount ___ Time of day ___	No Exercise ___ Morning ___ Afternoon ___ Evening ___ 2–3 hrs before bed	Names of medications	Shower/Bath ___ A.M./P.M. Nap (accidentally fell asleep) ___ A.M./P.M.
Day 7	1 = extremely 2 = sort of sleepy 3 = not at all	___ Yes ___ No Where?	___ Yes ___ No Nap 1: Length ___ min. Where? Nap 2: Length ___ min. Where? Nap 3: Length ___ min. Where?	Had no caffeine ___ Type and amount ___ Time of day ___ Type and amount ___ Time of day ___ Type and amount ___ Time of day ___	No Exercise ___ Morning ___ Afternoon ___ Evening ___ 2–3 hrs before bed	Names of medications	Shower/Bath ___ A.M./P.M. Nap (accidentally fell asleep) ___ A.M./P.M.

MORNING DIARY

Day/Date	About 1 hour before bed, my main activity was	What time did I get into bed last night?	How long did it take me to fall asleep last night?	How many times did I awaken in the middle of the night?	Total time spent awake during the night	My sleep was disturbed by	What time did I get out of bed this morning?	Total amount of sleep	What woke me up this morning?
Day 1		——— A.M./P.M.	——— Minutes	——— 0 ——— 1 ——— 2 ——— 3	——— Minutes	——— Noise ——— Stress ——— Need to use bathroom ——— Body aches ——— Temperature (too hot or cold) ——— Other	——— A.M./P.M.	——— Hours ——— Minutes	——— Alarm ——— Noise ——— Woke on my own Other: ———
Day 2		——— A.M./P.M.	——— Minutes	——— 0 ——— 1 ——— 2 ——— 3	——— Minutes	——— Noise ——— Stress ——— Need to use bathroom ——— Body aches ——— Temperature (too hot or cold) ——— Other	——— A.M./P.M.	——— Hours ——— Minutes	——— Alarm ——— Noise ——— Woke on my own Other: ———
Day 3		——— A.M./P.M.	——— Minutes	——— 0 ——— 1 ——— 2 ——— 3	——— Minutes	——— Noise ——— Stress ——— Need to use bathroom ——— Body aches ——— Temperature (too hot or cold) ——— Other	——— A.M./P.M.	——— Hours ——— Minutes	——— Alarm ——— Noise ——— Woke on my own Other: ———

	A.M./P.M.	Minutes	0 1 2 3	Minutes	Noise / Stress / Need to use bathroom / Body aches / Temperature (too hot or cold) / Other	A.M./P.M.	Hours / Minutes	Alarm / Noise / Woke on my own / Other:
Day 4	A.M./P.M.	Minutes	0 1 2 3	Minutes	Noise / Stress / Need to use bathroom / Body aches / Temperature (too hot or cold) / Other	A.M./P.M.	Hours / Minutes	Alarm / Noise / Woke on my own / Other:
Day 5	A.M./P.M.	Minutes	0 1 2 3	Minutes	Noise / Stress / Need to use bathroom / Body aches / Temperature (too hot or cold) / Other	A.M./P.M.	Hours / Minutes	Alarm / Noise / Woke on my own / Other:
Day 6	A.M./P.M.	Minutes	0 1 2 3	Minutes	Noise / Stress / Need to use bathroom / Body aches / Temperature (too hot or cold) / Other	A.M./P.M.	Hours / Minutes	Alarm / Noise / Woke on my own / Other:
Day 7	A.M./P.M.	Minutes	0 1 2 3	Minutes	Noise / Stress / Need to use bathroom / Body aches / Temperature (too hot or cold) / Other	A.M./P.M.	Hours / Minutes	Alarm / Noise / Woke on my own / Other:

Part II: Health and Sleep Habits Questionnaire

Adapted from Wolfson and Carkasdon 1998; Wolfson and Anwer 2000

Women's Health and Sleep Habits Questionnaire

Instructions

Answer the questions on the following pages as accurately and honestly as you can. There are no right or wrong answers.

* Do not spend too much time on one answer. Your first impression is usually best.

* Answer each question in the order that it appears. Try to answer all questions.

Section 1: Background Information and Work Schedule

Your age: _____

1. What is the status of your current employment? (Check all that apply.)

_____ a. Working full-time

_____ b. Working part-time

_____ c. Home keeper

_____ d. On maternity leave and returning

_____ e. On maternity leave and not returning to work

_____ f. Unemployed; looking for work

_____ g. Unemployed; not looking for work

_____ h. Student

_____ i. Retired

_____ j. Unable to work because _____

2. a. What hours do you work and/or attend school? (check all that apply) (write in specific time)

_____ a. Daytime

_____ b. Evening

_____ c. Weekdays

_____ d. Weekends

_____ e. Full-time

_____ f. Part-time

b. During your last work/school week, how many hours did you work, attend school, and/or do school work?

At your workplace or school: _____ hours

At home: _____ hours

c. During the last week, how many hours did you spend caring for your family and your home?

_____ hours

3. Who in you home is responsible for household chores and responsibilities (i.e., housecleaning)?

_____ a. I am

_____ b. My spouse/partner is

_____ c. My spouse/partner and I share responsibilities equally

_____ d. My spouse/partner helps

_____ e. Hired help

_____ f. Other: _____

4. What is the status of your spouse/partner's employment?(check all that apply)

_____ a. Working full-time

_____ b. Working part-time

_____ c. Home keeper

_____ d. On maternity leave and returning

_____ e. On maternity leave and not returning to work

_____ f. Unemployed; looking for work

_____ g. Unemployed; not looking for work

_____ h. Student

_____ i. Retired

_____ j. Unable to work because _____

5. a. What hours does your spouse/partner work and/or attend school? (check all that apply)(write in specific time)

_____ a. Daytime

_____ b. Evening

_____ c. Weekdays

_____ d. Weekends

_____ e. Full-time

_____ f. Part-time

b. According to your last work/school week, how many hours did your spouse/partner work and/or attend school?

At his/her workplace or school: _____ hours

At home: _____ hours

c. According to your last week, how many hours did your spouse/partner spend caring for your family and your home?

_____ hours

Section II: General Health Information

In the past two weeks, have you experienced any of the following conditions?

	Yes	No	Don't know	Comments:
a. Colds or flu?				
b. Increased difficulty breathing when suffering from colds or flu?	—	—	—	_____
c. Frequent nausea/vomiting?	—	—	—	_____
d. Poor appetite?	—	—	—	_____
e. Difficulty swallowing?	—	—	—	_____
f. Hearing problems?	—	—	—	_____
g. Speech problems?	—	—	—	_____
h. Ear infections?	—	—	—	_____
i. Nasal allergies or runny nose?	—	—	—	_____

7. In the past two weeks, how often did you participate in physical exercise (e.g., walking, jogging, biking, swimming)?

_____ a. Not at all

_____ b. Once a week

_____ c. Two or three times a week

_____ d. More than three times a week

If you did not exercise, skip to question 12.

8. How long have you been participating in regular physical activity?

_____ a. Longer than a month

_____ b. Longer than three months

_____ c. Longer than six months

_____ d. Longer than a year

9. How many hours did you exercise or work out per session in the last two weeks?

_____ a. 15–30 minutes

_____ b. 30–45 minutes

_____ c. 45–60 minutes

_____ d. over an hour

10. What time of day did you exercise in the last two weeks?

_____ a. Morning before work, between 5:00 and 9:00 A.M.

_____ b. Mid-morning, between 9:00 A.M. and 12:00 noon

_____ c. Afternoon, between noon and 3:00 P.M.

_____ d. Late afternoon, between 3:00 and 6:00 P.M.

_____ e. Evening, between 6:00 and 9:00 P.M.

_____ f. Late evening, after 9:00 P.M.

11. If you do exercise, how and to what extent did the exercise affect your sleep? (Check all that apply.)

_____ a. Made it easier to fall asleep

_____ b. Made it more difficult to fall asleep

_____ c. Made no difference when falling asleep

_____ d. Made it easier to get up in the morning

_____ e. Made it more difficult to get up in the morning

_____ f. Made no difference in getting up in the morning

_____ g. Made you more alert during the day

_____ h. Made you less alert during the day

_____ i. Made no difference during the day

Section III: Sleep/Wake Habits

12. In the last two weeks, what time did you usually go to bed on weekdays? (List ONE time, not a range.)

_____ : _____ A.M./P.M.

13. There are many reasons for doing things at one time or another. What is the main reason you usually go to bed at this time on weekdays? (Check one.)

_____ a. I feel sleepy.

_____ b. I am bored.

_____ c. My TV shows are over.

_____ d. I finish my office work.

_____ e. I finish my housework.

_____ f. My spouse goes to bed.

_____ g. I finish socializing/talking on phone.

_____ h. I get home from my job.

_____ i. Other: _____

14. In the last two weeks, what time did you usually wake up on weekdays? (List ONE time, not a range.)

    _____:_____ A.M./P.M.

15. What is the main reason you usually wake up at this time on weekdays? (Check one.)

    _____ a. My child or my pet wakes me up.

    _____ b. My alarm clock wakes me up.

    _____ c. My spouse wakes me up.

    _____ d. I need to go to the bathroom.

    _____ e. Pregnancy symptoms wake me up.

    _____ f. I don't know—I just wake up.

    _____ g. Other: _____

16. How long do you usually sleep on a normal weeknight?. (Do not include the time you spend awake in bed.)

    _____ hours _____ minutes

17. On weeknights, after you go to bed, about how long does it take you to fall asleep?

    _____ minutes

18. In the last two weeks, what time do you usually go to bed on weekends? (List ONE time, not a range.)

    _____:_____ A.M./P.M.

19. There are many reasons for doing things at one time or another. What is the main reason you usually go to bed at this time on weekends? (Check one.)

    _____ a. I feel sleepy.

    _____ b. I am bored.

    _____ c. My TV shows are over.

    _____ d. I finish my office work.

    _____ e. I finish my housework.

    _____ f. My spouse goes to bed.

    _____ g. I finish socializing/talking on phone.

    _____ h. I get home from my job.

    _____ i. Other: _____

20. In the last two weeks, what time did you usually wake up on weekends? (List ONE time, not a range.)

    _____ : _____ A.M./P.M.

21. What is the main reason you usually wake up at this time on weekends? (choose one)

    _____ a. My child or my pet wakes me up.

    _____ b. My alarm clock wakes me up.

    _____ c. My spouse wakes me up.

    _____ d. I need to go to the bathroom.

    _____ e. Pregnancy symptoms wake me up.

    _____ f. I don't know—I just wake up.

    _____ g. Other: _____

22. How long do you usually sleep on a night when you do not have to work the next day (such as a weekend night)? (Do not include the time you spend awake in bed.)

    _____ hours _____ minutes

23. On weekends, after you go to bed at night, about how long does it take you to fall asleep?

    _____ minutes

24. Some people wake up during the night: others never do. In the last two weeks, did you wake up in the middle of the night? _____ Yes _____ No

    If yes: on average, how many times a night did you wake up? _____ times

    How many nights a week did you wake up during the night?

    _____

    On average, how long did you remain awake? _____

25. Some people take naps in the daytime every day; others never do. In the last two weeks, did you take naps? _____ Yes _____ No

    If yes, how many times did you nap per day? _____

    How many times per week? _____

    How long did these naps usually last? _____ minutes

26. Do you know how much sleep you need? Fill out below how much sleep you think you would need each night to feel your best every day. (Do not include time you spend awake in bed.)

    _____ hours _____ minutes

27. In the last two weeks, what has been your usual sleeping position? (Check one.)

_____ a. on back

_____ b. on side

_____ c. on abdomen

_____ d. propped up/sitting

28. Have you been a restless sleeper during the past two weeks?
_____ Yes _____ No

29. Have you had a problem with falling asleep in the past two weeks?

_____ a. No

_____ b. Yes, mild

_____ c. Yes, moderate

_____ d. Yes, severe

30. In the last two weeks, how often have you had an unpleasant feeling in your legs at night (not leg cramps), such as creeping, crawling, or aching feelings that cause you to feel as if you need to move your legs?

_____ a. almost every night

_____ b. at least one week

_____ c. less than once a week

_____ d. less than once every two weeks

_____ e. never

Is this feeling relieved by moving your legs? _____ Yes _____ No

How distressing is this situation?

_____ a. not distressing

_____ b. mildly distressing

_____ c. moderately distressing

_____ d. severely distressing

How long do these sensations usually last?

_____ a. a few seconds

_____ b. less than 30 minutes

_____ c. more than 30 minutes, less than 1 hour

_____ d. more than 1 hour

31. Have you had a problem with waking up too early in the morning in the past two weeks? _____ Yes _____ No

32. How would you rate your sleep?
   ____ a. highly unsatisfactory
   ____ b. unsatisfactory
   ____ c. neither satisfactory or unsatisfactory
   ____ d. satisfactory
   ____ e. highly satisfactory

33. During the last two weeks, how often did you (mark one answer for each item):
   A=Not at all   B=Once   C=More than once but not every day D=Every day

	A	B	C	D
a. drink soda with caffeine?	__	__	__	__
b. drink coffee or tea with caffeine?	__	__	__	__
c. use tobacco (cigarettes, cigars, or chewing tobacco)?	__	__	__	__
d. drink alcohol (beer, wine, or liquor)?	__	__	__	__
e. use drugs (e.g., marijuana or cocaine)? Specify type: _____	__	__	__	__
f. use medications to help you sleep (prescription, nonprescription, or over-the-counter) Specify type: _____	__	__	__	__

Part III: Exercise Record

From Mary Ellen Copeland, *The Depression Workbook* (Oakland, Calif.: New Harbinger Publications, 1992): Copy this chart into a notebook to keep track of your daily exercise program.

Daily Exercise Record Week of:				
Date	How long I exercised	Type of exercise	How I felt before	How I felt afterward

Part IV: Relaxation Training

Adapted from *The Relaxation & Stress Reduction Workbook, 5th edition* and *The Anxiety & Phobia Workbook, 3rd edition* (Oakland, Calif.: New Harbinger Publications, 2000)

Background

Applied relaxation training brings together a number of proven relaxation techniques. The combined effect is both rapid and powerful, helping you reverse the effects of high stress in under a minute. Since the program is progressive, you will be adding new features to the exercise over the course of several weeks, while taking away other features once they have become habitual. Eventually you will be able to achieve deep relaxation in twenty to thirty seconds, quickly calming both your body and your mind when you encounter a stressful situation.

Applied relaxation can be helpful in a variety of life situations, from daily fights and frustrations to difficulty falling asleep at night.

In general, the program teaches you to relax by using a physical-relaxation process. You then progress to a conditioned relaxation response and finally learn to relax on command. You will also progress from practicing in a relaxed exercise setting to using the technique in real-life situations.

Symptom Effectiveness

Although applied relaxation was developed to treat individuals with phobias, it has a wide range of applications in other areas, including panic disorder, generalized anxiety disorder, sleep-onset insomnia, headache (e.g., tension, migraine), and back and joint pain.

Time to Master

You will notice some relaxation after just one or two sessions of relaxation training. Remember that this a progressive program. Each new stage will help you relax more quickly and more deeply, until you can relax at will in less than a minute. Do not rush yourself. You'll want to master each step of the program before you move on to the next step. Allow yourself one to two weeks, with two practice sessions a day, to feel comfortable with each step. If this sounds like a lot of time, keep in mind that your practice sessions can become the most refreshing part of your day. You can expect to spend approximately five to eight weeks progressing through the program.

Instructions

Applied relaxation training involves learning five separate stages. Each stage builds on the one before it, so be sure to follow all five stages in their listed order. You may find it useful to record a tape to guide yourself through the exercises that follow. A tape will help you focus your body and free you to close your eyes. To make a tape, use the instructions for each step as your script. Speak in a slow, even voice and be sure not to rush through the process.

Progressive Muscle Relaxation

Adapted from *The Anxiety & Phobia Workbook, 3rd edition*

Progressive muscle relaxation will help you recognize the difference between tension and relaxation in each of the major muscle groups. Surprising as it may sound, these distinctions are easy to overlook. Once you can really feel the difference between a tense muscle and a deeply relaxed one, you will be able to identify your chronic trouble spots and consciously rid them of their locked-in tension. You will also be able to bring your muscles to a deeper state of relaxation after you relax them than you could have if you hadn't tensed them first. Give yourself one to two weeks to master the technique, with two fifteen-minute practice sessions per day. Your goal should be to relax your entire body in one fifteen-to-twenty-minute session.

Progressive muscle relaxation is a systematic technique for achieving a deep state of relaxation. It was developed by Dr. Edmund Jacobson more than fifty years ago. Dr. Jacobson discovered that a muscle could be relaxed by first tensing it for a few seconds and then releasing it. Tensing and releasing various muscle groups throughout the body produces a deep state of relaxation, which Dr. Jacobson found capable of relieving a variety of conditions, from high blood pressure to ulcerative colitis.

In his original book, *Progressive Relaxation*, Dr. Jacobson developed a series of 200 different muscle relaxation exercises and a training program that took months to complete. More recently the system has been abbreviated to fifteen to twenty basic exercises, which have been found to be just as effective, if practiced regularly, as the original more elaborate system.

Progressive muscle relaxation is especially helpful for people whose anxiety is strongly associated with muscle tension. This is what often leads you to say that you are "uptight" or "tense." You may experience chronic tightness in your shoulders and neck, which can be effectively relieved by practicing progressive muscle relaxation. Other symptoms that respond well to progressive muscle relaxation include tension headaches, backaches, tightness in jaw, tightness around the eyes, muscle spasms, high blood pressure, and insomnia. If you are troubled by racing thoughts, you may find that systematically relaxing your muscles tends to help slow down your mind.

Long-term effects of *regular* practice of progressive muscle relaxation include

* A reduction in the time that it takes to fall asleep at night

* A decrease in generalized anxiety

* A decrease in anticipatory anxiety related to phobias

* Reduction in the frequency and duration of panic attacks

* Improved ability to face phobic situations through graded exposure

* Improved concentration

* An increased sense of control over moods

* Increased self-esteem

The *regular* practice of progressive muscle relaxation can go a long way toward helping you to better manage your anxiety, sleep difficulties, pain management, and to feel better all around. There are no contraindications for progressive muscle relaxation unless the muscle groups to be tensed and relaxed have been injured.

Guidelines for Practicing Progressive Muscle Relaxation

The following guidelines will help you make the most use of progressive muscle relaxation. They are also applicable to *any* form of deep relaxation you undertake to practice regularly, including self-hypnosis, guided visualization, and meditation.

1. Practice at least 20 *minutes per day*. Two 20-minute periods are preferable. Once a day is mandatory for obtaining generalized effects. (You may want to begin your practice with 30-minute periods. As you gain skill in relaxation technique, you will find that the amount of time you need to experience the relaxation response will decrease.)

2. Find a *quiet* location to practice where you won't be distracted. Don't permit the phone to ring while you're practicing. Use a fan or air conditioner to blot out background noise if necessary.

3. Practice at *regular times*. On awakening, before retiring, or before meals are generally the best times. A consistent daily relaxation routine will increase the likelihood of generalization effects.

4. Practice on *empty stomach*. Food digestion after meals will tend to disrupt your deep relaxation.

5. Assume a *comfortable position*. Your entire body, including your head, should be supported. Lying down on a sofa or bed or sitting in a reclining chair are two ways of supporting your body most completely. (When lying down, you may want to place a pillow beneath your knees for further support.) Sitting up is preferable to lying down if you are feeling tired and sleepy. It's advantageous to experience the full depth of the relaxation response consciously without going to sleep.

6. *Loosen any tight garments* and take off shoes, watch, glasses, contact lenses, jewelry, and so on.

7. Make a decision not to worry about anything. Give yourself permission to put aside the concerns of the day. Allow taking care of yourself and having peace of mind to take precedence over any of your worries. (Success with relaxation depends on giving peace of mind high priority in your overall scheme of values.)

8. Assume a *passive, detached attitude*. This is probably the most important element. You want to adopt a "let it happen" attitude and be free of any worry about how well you are performing the technique. Do not try to relax. Do not try to control your body. Do not judge your performance. The point is to let go.

Progressive Muscle Relaxation Technique

Progressive muscle relaxation involves tensing and relaxing, in succession, sixteen different muscle groups of the body. The idea is to tense each muscle group hard (not so hard that your muscles strain, however) for about ten seconds, and then to let go of it suddenly. You then give yourself fifteen to twenty seconds to relax, noticing how the muscle group feels when relaxed in contrast to how it feels when tensed, before going on to the next group of muscles. You might also say to yourself "I am relaxing," "Letting go," "Let the tension flow away," or any other relaxing phrase during each relaxation period between successive muscle groups. Throughout the exercise, maintain your focus on your muscles. When your attention wanders, bring it back to the particular muscle group you're working on. The guidelines below describes muscle relaxation in detail:

* Make sure you are in a setting that is quiet and comfortable. Observe the guidelines for practicing relaxation that were previously described.

* When you tense a particular muscle group, do so vigorously, without straining, for 7–10 seconds. You may want to count "one-thousand-one," "one-thousand-two," and so on, as a way of marking off seconds.

* Concentrate on what is happening. Feel the buildup of tension in each particular muscle group. It is often helpful to visualize the particular muscle group being tensed.

* When you release the muscles, do so abruptly, and then relax, enjoying the sudden feeling of limpness. Allow the relaxation to develop for at least 15–20 seconds before going on to the next group of muscles.

* Allow all the *other* muscles in your body to remain relaxed, as far as possible, while working on a particular muscle group.

* Tense and relax each muscle group once. But if a particular area feels especially tight, you can tense and relax it two or three times, waiting about 20 seconds between each cycle.

Once you are comfortably supported in a quiet place, followed the detailed instructions below:

1. To begin, take three deep abdominal breaths, exhaling slowly each time. As you exhale, imagine that tension throughout your body begins to flow away.

2. Clench your fists. Hold for 7–10 seconds and then release for 15–20 seconds. *Use these same time intervals for all other muscle groups.*

3. Tighten your biceps by drawing your forearms up toward your shoulders and "making a muscle" with both arms. Hold . . . and then relax.

4. Tighten your *triceps*—the muscles on the undersides of your upper arms—by extending your arms out straight and locking your elbows. Hold . . . and then relax.

5. Tense the muscles in your forehead by raising your eyebrows as far as you can. Hold . . . and then relax. Imagine your forehead muscles becoming smooth and limp as they relax.

6. Tense the muscles around your eyes by clenching your eyelids tightly shut. Hold . . . and then relax. Imagine sensations of deep relaxation spreading all around the area of your eyes.

7. Tighten your jaw by opening your mouth so widely that you stretch the muscles around the hinges of your jaw. Hold . . . and then relax. Let your lips part and allow your jaw to hang loose.

8. Tighten the muscles in the back of your neck by pulling your head way back, as if you were going to touch your head to your back (be gentle with this muscle group to avoid injury.) Focus only on tensing the muscles in your neck. Hold and then relax. Since this area is often especially tight, it's good to do the tense-relax cycle twice.

9. Take a few deep breaths and tune in to the weight of your head sinking into whatever surface it is resting on.

10. Tighten your shoulders by raising them up as if you were going to touch your ears. Hold . . . and then relax.

11. Tighten the muscles around your shoulder blades by pushing your shoulder blades back as if you were going to touch them together.

    Hold the tension in your shoulder blades . . . and then relax. Since this area is often especially tense, you might repeat the tense-relax sequence twice.

12. Tighten the muscles of your chest by taking in a deep breath. Hold for up to 10 seconds . . . and then release slowly. Imagine any excess tension in your chest flowing away with the exhalation.

13. Tighten your stomach muscles by sucking your stomach in. Hold . . . and then release. Imagine a wave of relaxation spreading through your abdomen.

14. Tighten your lower back by arching it up. (You can omit this exercise if you have lower back pain.) Hold . . . and then relax.

15. Tighten your buttocks by pulling them together. Hold . . . and then relax. Imagine the muscles in your hips going loose and limp.

16. Squeeze the muscles in your thighs all the way down to your knees. You will probably have to tighten your hips along with your thighs, since the thigh muscles attach at the pelvis. Hold . . . and then relax. Feel your thigh muscles smoothing out and relaxing completely.

17. Tighten your calf muscles by pulling your toes toward you (flex carefully to avoid cramps.) Hold . . . and then relax.

18. Tighten your feet by curling your toes downward. Hold . . . and then relax.

19. Mentally scan your body for any residual tension. If a particular area remains tense, repeat one or two tense-relax cycles for that group of muscles.

20. Now imagine a wave of relaxation slowly spreading throughout your body, starting at your head and gradually penetrating every muscle group all the way down to your toes.

The entire progressive muscle relaxation sequence should take you twenty to thirty minutes the first time. With practice you may decrease the time needed to fifteen to twenty minutes. You might want to record the above exercises on an audiocassette to expedite your early practice sessions. Or you may wish to obtain a professionally made tape of progressive muscle relaxation exercise. (See below.) Some people may always prefer to use a tape, while others have the exercises so well learned after a few weeks of practice that they prefer doing them from memory.

Remember, regular practice of progressive muscle relaxation once a day will produce a significant reduction in your overall level of anxiety. It will also reduce the frequency and intensity of panic attacks. Finally, regular practice will reduce anticipatory anxiety that may arise in the course of systematically exposing yourself to phobic situations, insomnia, and other anxiety-provoking situations.

Resources

The following audiotape for relaxation can be obtained from New Harbinger Publications by calling 1-800-748-6273.

P. Fanning, M. McKay, and N. Sonenberg. 1991. *Applied Relaxation Training*. Oakland, Calif.: New Harbinger Publications. (Item #24)

Part V: Migraine & Tension Headache Assessment

Adapted by permission of Richard B. Lipton, M.D., Professor of Neurology, Albert Einstein College of Medicine, New York, NY, and Walter F. Stewart, M.P.H., Ph.D., Associate Professor of Epidemiology, John Hopkins University, Baltimore, MD. [Stewart et al., published in *Neurology* 53(5), 988–994].

These questions were put together to help you measure the impact your headaches have had on your life over the last three months and to communicate this more effectively. The best way to measure this is by counting the numbers of days of your life which are affected by headaches. You can do this for yourself as follows:

For questions 1 and 2, **work or school** means paid work or education if you are student at a school or college. For questions 3 and 4, household work means activities such as housework, home repairs and maintenance, shopping as well as caring for children and relatives.

INSTRUCTIONS: Please answer the following questions about ALL your headaches you have had over the last three months. Put your answer next to each question. If a single headache affects more than one area of your life (e.g., work and family life) it should be counted more than once. If you did not have the activity in the last three months, put zero.

1. On how many days in the last 3 months did you miss work or school because of your headaches?

2. How many days in the last 3 months was your productivity at work or school reduced by half or more because of your headaches? (Do not include days you counted on question 1 where you missed work or school.)

3. On how many days in the last 3 months did you not do household work because of your headaches?

4. How many days in the last 3 months was your productivity in household work reduced by half or more because of your headaches? (Do not include days you counted in question 3 where you did not do household work.)

5. On how many days in the last 3 months did you miss family, social, or leisure activities because of your headaches?

6. On how many days in the last 3 months did you have a headache? (If a headache lasted more than 1 day, count each day.)

7. On a scale of 1–10, on average how painful were these headaches? (where 0 = no pain at all, and 10 = pain as bad as it can be.)

Part VI: Pain Diary

Adapted, with permission from Guilford Press, from Margaret A. Claudill, M.D., *Managing Pain Before It Manages You* (New York: Guilford Press, 1994)

Keeping a pain diary is an effective way to raise awareness of the triggers and consequences of your pain, and it is a first step toward taking control of your pain. The following is Dr. Caudill's "pain diary" method:

* Designate an actual diary or notebook for this purpose.

* Record your pain levels in the diary three times a day at regular time intervals (e.g., morning, noon, and bedtime).

* Describe the situation or activity that corresponds in time to each rating. For instance, were you working, watching TV, talking to a friend?

* Rate your pain sensations, which refers to the physical aspects of your pain, such as achiness, stabbing, burning, tightness, or other sensations:
0 = no pain; 1–9 = ranges in degree of pain; 10 = the worst possible distress.

* Also rate your pain distress, which refers to your perception of pain, and is a measure of the emotional suffering you experience, such as frustration, anger, anxiety, sadness, and so on: 0 = no distress; 1–9 = ranges in degree of distress; 10 = the worst possible distress.

Start by keeping this pain diary for one week, then analyze the results. Search for patterns associated with your pain. They may be simple physical associations, such as an increase in pain when you get up in the morning, start eating, and so on. Also notice any correlations between emotional states, stressful events, or certain relationships and the onset of pain.

Be on the lookout for discrepancies between your ratings of your pain sensations and pain distress. You may find, as many patients do—that your distress and numbers are frequently higher than your pain sensation numbers. What's the significance? It means that your pain perception, and your emotional suffering, go well beyond your physical sensations. At these times, your suffering about pain is a predominant factor in your pain experience. The purpose of the exercise is to separate your perceptions from your actual sensations, until you are fully aware of the gaps. When your pain sensations rate a three but your distress about pain is a seven, you know it is time to quiet your overanxious mind. When you do, it becomes easier to adopt thoughts such as: "Maybe I can live with this level of pain." "Perhaps by reducing my distress I can relieve some of my pain."

Emotional suffering around pain may feed back into pain processing centers in your nervous system, thus perpetuating your physical pain sensations. Therefore, it helps to remember that modifying your relentlessly negative thoughts and feelings about pain is one strategy to reduce pain itself!

* *

Appendix C

Resources

Chapter 1: Normal Sleep over the Life Span

Centers, Organizations, and Foundations:

American Academy of Sleep Medicine (AASM)
(Formerly known as American Sleep Disorders Association)
6301 Bandel Road NW, Suite 101
Rochester, MN 55901
Telephone: (507) 287-6006
Fax: (507) 287-6008
E-mail: info@aasmnet.org
Web site: www.aasmnet.org

The National Sleep Foundation (NSF)
1522 K Street NW, Suite 500
Washington, DC 20005
Telephone: (202) 785-2300
Fax: (202) 347-3472
E-mail: nsf@sleepfoundation.org
Web site: www.sleepfoundation.org

Recommended Reading:

Binkley, Sue. 1997. *Biological Clocks: Your Owner's Manual*. Newark, N.J.: Harwood Academic Publishers.

Dement, William C., and Christopher Vaughan. 2000. The Promise of Sleep. Toronto: Dell Books.

Hobson, Allan, J. 1995. *Sleep*. New York: W. H. Freeman & Company.

Kleitman, Nathaniel. 1987. *Sleep and Wakefulness*. Chicago: University of Chicago Press.

Kryger, Meir H., Thomas Roth, and William C. Dement. 2000. *Principle and Practice of Sleep Medicine*. Philadelphia: W. B. Saunders Company.

Chapter 2: Understanding Your Menstrual Cycle and Sleep Patterns

Web Sites:

Endometriosis.org
www.endometriosis.org

PeriodWatch.com
www.periodwatch.com

Centers, Organizations, Foundations:

Endometriosis Association International Headquarters
8585 North Seventy-sixth Place
Milwaukee, WI 53223
Telephone: (414) 355-2200; (800) 992-3636
Fax: (414) 355-6065
E-mail: endo@endometriosisassn.org
Web site: www.endometriosisassn.org

Endometriosis Institute
2425 West Twenty-second Street
Oak Brook, IL 60523
Telephone: (630) 954-0054
Fax: (630) 954-0064
Web site: www.endometriosisinstitute.com/

Endometriosis Research Center
630 Ibis Drive
Delray Beach, FL 33444
Telephone: (561) 274-7442; (800) 239-7280
Fax: (561) 274-9117
E-mail: EndoFL@aol.com
Web site: www.endocenter.org

National Women's Health Network
514 Tenth Street NW, Suite 400
Washington, DC 20004
Telephone: (202) 347-1140
Fax: (202) 347-1168.
Web site: www.womenshealthnetwork.org

Recommended Reading:

Ballweg, Mary Lou, Dan Martin, and Endometriosis Association. 1995. *The Endometriosis Sourcebook: The Definitive Guide to Current Treatment Options, the Latest Research, Common Myths About the Disease and Coping Strategies.* Lincolnwood, Ill.: NTC/Contemporary Publishing Group.

Dan, Alice J., and Linda L. Lewis. 1991. *Menstrual Health in Women's Lives.* Urbana, Ill.: University of Illinois Press.

Futterman, Lori, A.. 1998. *The PMS & Perimenopause Sourcebook: A Guide to the Emotional, Mental, and Physical Patterns of a Woman's Life.* Chicago: Lowell House.

Phillips, Robert H., and Glenda Motta. 2000. *Coping with Endometriosis: A Practical Guide to Understanding, Treating and Living with Chronic Endometriosis.* Garden City Park, N.Y.: Avery Publishing Group.

Walker, Anne E. 1997. *The Menstrual Cycle (Women and Psychology).* New York: Routledge.

Chapter 3: Sleep Patterns during Pregnancy

Web Sites:

BabyCenter
www.babycenter.com/pregnancysleep

Centers, Organizations, and Foundations:

The American College of Obstetricians and Gynecologists (ACOG)
P.O. Box 96920
Washington, DC 20090-6920
E-mail: Mark Graves, mgraves@acog.com
Web site: www.acog.com

Chapter 4: Childbirth and Postpartum Months: Sleeping for Two or More

Centers, Organizations, and Foundations"

Depression After Delivery
P.O. Box 278
Belle Mead, NJ 08502
Telephone: (908) 575-9121; (800) 944-4PPD (information request line)

Postpartum Support International
927 North Kellogg Avenue

Santa Barbara, CA 93111
Telephone: (805) 967-7636
Fax: (805) 967-0608
E-mail: jhonikman@earthlink.net
Web site: www.postpartum.net

Recommended Reading:

Cuthbertson, Joanne, and Susie Schevill. 1985. *Helping Your Child Sleep Through the Night*. New York: Doubleday.

Ferber, Richard. 1986. *Solve Your Child's Sleep Problems*. New York: Simon & Schuster.

Mindell, Jodi A. 1997. *Sleeping Through the Night: How Infants, Toddlers, and Their Parents Can Get a Good Night's Sleep*. New York: HarperCollins.

Nicolson, Paula. 1998. *Post-Natal Depression: Psychology, Science and the Transition to Motherhood (Women and Psychology)*. New York: Routledge.

Chapter 5: Sleep-Wake Patterns during Menopause

Web Sites:

Menopause Online
www.menopause-online.com
info@menopause-online.com

The Mid-Life and Menopause Support Group
www.span.com.au/midlife/index.html

Centers, Organizations, and Foundations:

North American Menopause Society
P.O. Box 94527
Cleveland, OH 44101-4527
Telephone: (444) 442-7550
Fax: (444) 442-2660
Web site: www.menopause.org

Recommended Reading:

American Medical Association. 1998. *AMA Essential Guide to Menopause*. New York: Pocket Books.

Huston, James E., M.D., and L. Darlene Lanka, M.D. 2000. *Perimenopause*. Second edition. Oakland, Calif.: New Harbinger Publications.

Chapter 6: Work, Motherhood, and Sleep

Centers, Organizations, and Foundations:

Catalyst
120 Wall Street
New York, NY 10005
Telephone: (212) 514-7600
Fax: (212) 514-8470
Web site: www.catalystwomen.org

National Partnership for Women & Families
1875 Connecticut Avenue NW, Suite 710
Washington, DC 20009
Telephone: (202) 986-2600
Fax: (202) 986-2539
E-mail: info@nationalpartnership.org
Web site: www.nationalpartnership.org

U.S. Department of Labor, Women's Bureau
200 Constitution Avenue NW, Room no. S-3002
Washington, DC 20210
Telephone: (800) 827-5335
Fax: (202) 219-5529
Web site: www.dol.gov/dol/wb

Women Employed
111 North Wabash, Floor 13
Chicago, IL 60602
Telephone: (312) 782-3902
Fax: (312) 782-5249
E-mail: info@womenemployed.org
Web site: www.womenemployed.org

Recommended Reading:

Barnett, Rosalind C., and Caryl Rivers. 1998. *She Works/He Works: How Two-Income Families Are Happy, Healthy, and Thriving*. Cambridge: Harvard University Press.

Chira, Susan. 1999. *A Mother's Place: Choosing Work and Family Without Guilt or Blame*. New York: HarperCollins.

Engberg, Karen. 1999. *It's Not the Glass Ceiling, It's the Sticky Floor: And Other Things Our Daughters Should Know About Marriage, Work, and Motherhood*. Amherst, N.Y.: Prometheus Books.

Harvard Business Review. 2000. *Harvard Business Review on Work and Life Balance*. Watertown, Mass.: Harvard Business School Press.

Monk, Timothy H., and Simon Folkard. 1992. *Making Shiftwork Tolerable*. New York: Taylor & Francis Group.

Chapter 7: Sleep Problems for Women: Insomnia

Web Sites:

Sleep Home Pages
www.sleephomepages.org

Sleep Medicine
http://sleepmed.bsd.uchicago.edu

Sleep Medicine Home Page
www.users.cloud9.net/~thorpy

Sleepnet.com
www.sleepnet.com/disorder.htm#sleep1

Sleep Research Society
www.srssleep.org

The Sleep Well
www.stanford.edu/~dement/

Centers, Organizations, and Foundations:

National Center on Sleep Disorders Research (NCSDR)
Two Rockledge Center
Suite 7024
6701 Rockledge Drive, MSC 7920
Bethesda, MD 20892-7920
Telephone: (301) 435-0199
Fax: (301) 480-3451
Web site: www.nhlbi.nih.gov/about/ncsdr/index.htm

Recommended Reading:

Hauri, Peter, Shirley Linde, and Philip Westbrook. 1996. *No More Sleepless Nights*. New York: John Wiley & Sons.

Jacobs, Gregg D., and Herbert Benson. 1999. *Say Goodnight to Insomnia*. Bellingham, Wash.: Owl Books.

Lichstein, Kenneth L., and Charles M. Morin. 2000. *Treatment of Late-Life Insomnia*. Thousand Oaks, Calif.: Sage Publications.

Morin, Charles M. 1996. *Insomnia: Psychological Assessment and Management*. New York: Guilford Publications.

———. 1996. *Relief from Insomnia: Getting the Sleep of Your Dreams*. New York: Doubleday Books.

Pressman, Mark R., and William C. Orr. 1997. *Understanding Sleep: The Evaluation and Treatment of Disorders*. Washington, D.C.: American Psychological Association.

Wiedman, John. 1999. *Desperately Seeking Snoozin'*. Memphis: Towering Pines Press.

Zammit, Gary K. 1998. *Good Nights: How to Stop Sleep Deprivation, Overcome Insomnia, and Get the Sleep You Need*. Kansas City, Mo.: Andrews McMeel Publishing.

Chapter 8: Sleep Apnea and Other Sleep Disorders

Centers, Organizations, and Foundations:

American Sleep Apnea Association
424 K Street NW, Suite 302
Washington, DC 20005
Telephone: (202) 293-3650
Fax: (202) 293-3656
E-mail: asaa@sleepapnea.org

Recommended Reading:

Pascualy, Ralph A. 2000. *Snoring and Sleep Apnea: Sleep Well, Feel Better*. New York: Demos.

Simpson, Carolyn. 1996. *Coping with Sleep Disorders*. New York: Rosen Publishing Group.

Swanson, Jennifer. 1999. *Sleep Disorders Sourcebook: Basic Consumer Health Information About Sleep and Its Disorders, Including Insomnia, Sleepwalking, Sleep Apnea, Restless Leg Syndrome, and Narcolepsy*. Detroit: Omnigraphics.

Chapter 9: Physical Health and Sleep

Web Sites:

Journal of the American Medical Association, Migraine Information Center
http://www.ama-assn.org/special/migraine/migraine.htm

National Fibromyalgia Research Association
http://www.teleport.com/~nfra

The National Women's Health Information Center
www.4woman.gov

MigrainePage.com
www.migrainepage.com

Centers, Organizations, and Foundations:

Association for the Advancement of Behavior Therapy
305 Seventh Avenue, Floor 16
New York, NY 10001-60008
Telephone: (212) 647-1890
Fax: (212) 647-1865
Web site: www.aabt.org

The American Institute for Cognitive Therapy (AICT)
136 East Fifty-seventh Street, Suite 1101
New York, NY 10022
Telephone: (212) 308-2440
E-mail: AICT@aol.com
Web site: www.cognitivetherapynyc.com/

American Medical Women's Association (AMWA)
801 North Fairfax Street, Suite 400
Alexandria, VA 22314
Telephone: (708) 838-0500
Fax: (703) 549-3864
E-mail: info@amwa-doc.org
Web site: www.amwa-doc.org

The Beck Institute for Cognitive Therapy and Research
GSB Building, City Line and Belmont Avenues, Suite 700
Bala Cynwyd, PA 19004-1610
Telephone: (610) 664-3020
Fax: (610) 664-4437
E-mail: beckinst@gim.net
Web site: www.beckinstitute.org/

Fibromyalgia Network
P.O. Box 31750
Tuscon, AZ 85751-1750
Telephone: (800) 853-2929
Web site: www.fmnetnews.com

Migraine Awareness Group, A National Understanding for
Migraineurs (M.A.G.N.U.M., INC.)
113 South Saint Asaph, Suite 300
Alexandria, VA 22314
Telephone: (703) 739-9384
Fax: (703) 739-2432
Web site: www.migraine.org

National Headache Foundation
428 West Saint James Place, Floor 2
Chicago, IL 60614-2750

Telephone: (888) NHF-5552; (773) 388-6399; (800) 843-2256 (headache hotline)
Fax: (773) 525-7357
E-mail: info@headaches.org
Web site: www.headaches.org/

National Institutes of Health Office of Research on Women's Health
Building 1, Room 201
9000 Rockville Pike
Bethesda, MD 20892
Telephone: (310) 402-1770

National Women's Health Resource Center
5255 Loughboro Road NW
Washington, DC 20016
Telephone: (202) 537-4015
Fax: (202) 778-6306
Web site: www.healthywomen.org

Society for Women's Health Research
1828 L Street NW, Suite 625
Washington, DC 20036
Telephone: (202) 223-8224
Fax: (202) 833-3472
Web site: www.womens-health.org

Recommended Reading:

Beck, Judith, and Aaron Beck. 1995. *Cognitive Therapy: Basics and Beyond*. New York: Guilford Press.

Bic, Zuzana, Frances Bic, and L. Francis Bic. 1999. *No More Headaches, No More Migraines*. New York: Avery Penguin Putnam.

Boston Women's Health Book Collective. 1998. *Our Bodies, Ourselves for the New Century: A Book by and for Women*. New York: Simon and Schuster.

Casper, Regina C. 1998. *Women's Health: Hormones, Emotions, and Behavior*. New York: Cambridge University Press.

Dement, William C., and Christopher Vaughan. 1999. *The Promise of Sleep: A Pioneer in Sleep Medicine Explains the Vital Connection Between Health, Happiness, and a Good Night's Sleep*. New York: Delacorte Press.

Domar, Alice D. 1997. *Healing Mind, Healthy Woman: Using the Mind-Body Connection to Manage Stress and Take Control of Your Life*. New York: Dell Publishing.

Peterson, Christina, and Christine Adamec. 1999. *The Women's Migraine Survival Guide: The Most Complete, Up-to-Date Resource on the Causes of Your Migraine Pain—And Treatments for Real Relief.* New York: Harperperennial Library.

Robbins, Jim. 2000. *A Symphony in the Brain: The Evolution of the New Brain Wave Biofeedback.* Boston: Atlantic Monthly Press.

St. Amand, R. Paul, and Claudia Craig Marek. 1999. *What Your Doctor May Not Tell You about Fibromyalgia: The Revolutionary Treatment That Can Reverse the Disease.* New York: Warner Books.

Schwartz, Mark S., and Frank Andrasik. 1998. *Biofeedback: A Practitioner's Guide.* New York: Guilford Press.

Starlanyl, Devin J., and Mary Ellen Copeland. 1996. *Fibromyalgia & Chronic Myofascial Pain Syndrome: A Survival Manual.* Oakland, Calif.: New Harbinger Publications.

―――. 1998. *Fibromyalgia Advocate: Getting the Support You Need to Cope with Fibromyalgia and Myofascial Pain Syndrome.* Oakland, Calif.: New Harbinger Publications.

Chapter 10: Emotional Well-Being and Sleep

Centers, Organizations, and Foundations:

American Psychiatric Association
1400 K Street NW
Washington, DC 20005
Telephone: (202) 682-6000
Fax: (202) 682-6850
Web site: www.psych.org

American Psychological Association
750 First Street NE
Washington, DC 20002-4242
Telephone: (800) 374-2721; (202) 336-5500
Web site: www.apa.org

Anxiety Disorders Association of America
11900 Parklawn Drive, Suite 100
Rockville, MD 20852
Web site: www.adaa.org

National Alliance for the Mentally Ill
3 Colonial Place
2107 Wilson Blvd., Suite 300
Arlington, VA 22201-3042
Telephone: (703) 524-7600; (800) 950-NAMI (help line)

Fax: (703) 524-9094

Web site: www.nami.org

National Depressive and Manic-Depressive Association
730 North Franklin Street, Suite 501
Chicago, Illinois 60610-3526
Telephone: (800) 826-3632; (312) 642-0049
Fax: (312) 642-7243
Web site: www.ndmda.org

National Foundation for Depressive Illness, Inc.
P.O. Box 2257
New York, NY 10116-2257
Telephone: (800) 239-1265
Web site: www.depression.org

National Institute of Mental Health (NIMH)
NIMH Public Inquiries
6001 Executive Boulevard, Room 8184, MSC 9663
Bethesda, MD 20892-9663
Telephone: (301) 443-4513
Fax: (301) 443-4279
Web site: www.nimh.nih.gov

National Mental Health Information Center
1020 Prince Street
Alexandria, VA 23314-2971
Telephone: (800) 969-6642

Recommended Reading:

DeRosis, Helen. 1998. *Women and Anxiety: A Step-By-Step Program for Managing Anxiety and Depression*. New York: Hatherleigh Press.

Jack, Dana Crowly. 1993. *Silencing the Self: Women and Depression*. New York: HarperCollins.

Nolen-Hoeksema, Susan. 1990. *Sex Differences in Depression*. Stanford, Calif.: Stanford University Press.

Steiner, Meir. 1998. *Depression in Women: Mood Disorders Associated With Reproductive Cyclicity*. London: Martin Dunitz.

References

Adair, R., H. Bauchner, B. Philipp, S. Levenson, and B. Zuckerman. 1991. Night waking during infancy: Role of parental presence at bedtime. *Pediatrics* 87:500–4.

Adair, R., B. Zuckerman, H. Bauchner, B. Philipp, and S. Levenson. 1992. Reducing night waking in infancy: A primary care intervention. *Pediatrics* 89:585–88.

Aldrich, M. S., and J. E. Shipley. 1993. Alcohol use and periodic limb movements in sleep. *Alcohol Clinical Experimental Research,* 171:192–196.

Alward, R. R., and T. H. Monk. 1990. A comparison of rotating shift and permanent night nurses. *International Journal of Nursing Studies* 27(3):297–302.

American Psychiatric Association. 1994. *Diagnostic and Statistical Manual of Mental Disorders.* Washington, D.C.: American Psychiatric Association.

Ancoli-Israel, S. 1996. *All I Want Is a Good Night's Sleep.* Boston: Mosby-Year Books.

Ancoli-Israel, S., D. F. Kripke, M. R. Klauber, W. J. Mason, R. Fell, and O. Kaplan. 1991. Periodic limb movements in sleep in community-dwelling elderly. *Sleep* 14:496–500.

Anders, T., and M. Keener. 1985. Developmental course of nighttime sleep-wake patterns in full-term and premature infants during the first year of life. *Sleep* 8(3):173–92.

Anthony, C.W., and W. A. Anthony. 1999. *The Art of Napping at Work.* New York: Larson Publications.

Baker, A., S. Simpson, and D. Dawson. 1997. Sleep disruption and mood changes associated with menopause. *Journal of Psychosomatic Research* 43(4):359-69.

Barlow, D. H. 1988. *Anxiety and Its Disorders: The Nature and Treatment of Anxiety and Panic.* New York: Guilford Press.

Barnett, R. C., and C. Rivers. 1996. *She Works/He Works: How Two-Income Families Are Happier, Healthier, and Better-Off.* San Francisco: Harper.

Barnett, R., Davidson, and Marshall. 1991. Physical symptoms and the interplay of work and family roles. *Health Psychology* 10(2): 94–101.

Bassett J., J. Giovanni, K. Peterson, K. McGurn, S. Trentacoste, A. Wolfson, and U. Anwer. 1999. Sleep and mood from the last trimester of pregnancy through four months postpartum. *Sleep* 22 (Supplement):245.

Beck, A., J. Rush, B. Shaw, and G. Emery. 1979. *The Cognitive Therapy of Depression.* New York: Guilford Press.

Benca, R. 2000. Mood disorders. In *Principles and Practice of Sleep Medicine,* edited by M. H. Kryger, T. Roth, and W. C. Dement. Philadelphia: Saunders.

Blehar, M. C., and D. A. Oren. 1995. Women's increased vulnerability to mood disorders: Integrating psychobiology and epidemiology. *Depression* 3:3–12.

Bliwise, D. L. 1991. Treating insomnia: Pharmacological and nonphar- macological approaches. *Journal of Psychoactive Drugs* 23(4):335–41.

Block, A. J., C. M. Bush, C. White, P. G. Boysen, J. W. Wynne, and V. C. Taasan. 1981. A radiographic method for measuring steady-state functional residual capacity in the supine patient. A method suitable for sleep studies. *The American Review of Respiratory Disease* 24(3):330–32.

Bootzin, R. R., D. Epstein, D., and J. M. Wood. 1991. Stimulus control instructions. In *Case Studies in Insomnia,* edited by P. J. Hauri. New York: Plenum Press.

Bootzin, R. R., and S. P. Rider. 1997. Behavioral techniques and biofeedback for insomnia. In *Understanding Sleep: The Evaluation and Treatment of Sleep Disorders,* edited by M. R. Pressman, and W. C. Orr. Washington, D.C.: APA.

Boston Women's Health Book Collective. 1998. *Our Bodies, Ourselves for the New Century: A Book by and for Women.* New York: Simon and Schuster.

Bourne, E. J. 2000. *The Anxiety and Phobia Workbook.* Oakland, Calif.: New Harbinger Publications.

Breslau, N., T. Roth, L. Rosenthal, and P. Andreski. 1996. Sleep disturbance and psychiatric disorders: A longitudinal epidemiological study of young adults. *Biological Psychiatry* 39:411–18.

Browman, C. P., M. G. Sampson, S. F. Yolles, K. S. Gujavarty, S. J. Weiler, J. A. Walsleben, P. M. Hahn, and M. M. Mitler. 1984. Obstructive sleep apnea and body weight. *Chest* 1982:291–94.

Brunello, N., R. Armitage, I. Feinberg, E. Holsboer-Trachsler, D. Leger, P. Linkowski, W. B. Mendelson, G. Racagni, B. Saletu, A. L. Sharpley, F. Turek, E. Van Cauter, and J. Mendlewicz. 2000. Depression and sleep disorders: Clinical relevance, economic burden and pharmacological treatment. *Biological Psychiatry* 42:107–19.

Burns, D. 1989. *The Feeling Good Handbook.* New York: William Morrow.

Burwell, C., E. Roben, R. Whaley, and A. Bikelman. 1956. Extreme obesity associated with alveolar hypoventilation: A Pickwickian syndrome. *American Journal of Medicine* 21:811–18.

Buskila, D., L. Neumann, I. Hazanov, and R. Carmi. 1996. Familial aggregation in the fibromyalgia syndrome. *Seminars in Arthritis Rheumatology* 26(3):605–11.

Buskila, D., L. Neumann, G. Vaisberg, D. Alkalay, and F. Wolfe. 1997. Increased rates of fibromyalgia following cervical spine injury. A controlled study of 161 cases of traumatic injury. *Arthritis Rheumatology* 40(3):446–52.

Carskadon, M. A. 1990. Patterns of sleep and sleepiness in adolescents. *Pediatrician* 17:5–12.

Carskadon, M. A., and W. C. Dement. 2000. Normal human sleep: An overview. In *Principles and Practice of Sleep Medicine,* edited by M. H. Kryger, T. Roth, and W. C. Dement. Philadelphia: Saunders.

Caudill, M. 1994. *Managing Pain Before It Manages You.* New York: Guilford Press.

Chesson, A., Jr., K. Hartse, W. M. Anderson, D. Davila, S. Johnson, M. Littner, M. Wise, J. Rafecas. 2000. Practice parameters for the evaluation of chronic insomnia. An American Academy of Sleep Medicine report. Standards of Practice Committee of the American Academy of Sleep Medicine. *Sleep* 23(2):237–41.

Clark, A. J., J. Flowers, L. Boots, and S. Shettar. 1995. Sleep disturbance in mid-life women. *Journal of Advanced Nursing* 22(3): 562–68.

Coates, T. J., and C. E. Thoresen. 1981. Sleep disturbance in children and adolescents. In *Behavioral Assessment of Childhood Disorders,* edited by E. G. Mash and L. G. Terdal. New York: Guilford Press.

Colditz, G. A., K. M. Egan, and M. J. Stampfer. 1993. Hormone replacement therapy and risk of breast cancer: Results from epidemiologic studies. *American Journal of Obstetrics and Gynecology* 168(5):1473–80.

Copeland, M. E., and M. McKay. 1992. *The Depression Workbook.* Oakland, Calif.: New Harbinger Publications.

Craske, M. G., and D. H. Barlow. 1989. Nocturnal panic. *Journal of Nervous and Mental Disease* 177:160–67.

Crowell, J., M. Keener, N. Ginsburg, and T. Anders. 1987. Sleep habits in toddlers eighteen to thirty-six months old. *Journal of American Academy of Child and Adolescent Psychiatry* 26:510–19.

Cuthbertson, J., and S. Schevill. 1985. *Helping Your Child Sleep Through the Night.* New York: Doubleday.

Czeisler, C.A., and S. B. S. Khalsa. 2000. The human circadian timing system and sleep-wake regulation. In *Principles and Practice of Sleep Medicine,* edited by M. H. Kryger, T. Roth, and W.C. Dement. Philadelphia, Pa.: Saunders.

Czeisler, C. A., G. S. Richardson, R. M. Coleman, J. C. Zimmerman, M. C. Moore-Ede, W. C. Dement, and E. D. Weitzman. 1981. Chronotherapy: Resetting the circadian clocks of patients with delayed sleep phase insomnia. *Sleep* 4:1–21.

Davis, M., E. R. Eshelman, and M. McKay. 2000. *The Relaxation and Stress Reduction Workbook.* Oakland, Calif.: New Harbinger Publications.

DiFranza, J. R., and R. A. Lew. 1995. Effect of maternal cigarette smoking on pregnancy complications and sudden infant death syndrome. *Journal of Family Practice* 40(4):385–94.

Domar, A. D., and H. Dreher. 1996. *Healing Mind, Healthy Woman: Using the Mind-Body Connection to Manage Stress and Take Control of Your Life.* New York: Dell Publishing.

Driver, H. S., and C. M. Shapiro. 1992. A longitudinal study of sleep stages in young women during pregnancy and postpartum. *Sleep* 15(5):449–53.

Driver, H. S., and F. C. Baker. 1998. Menstrual factors in sleep. *Sleep Medicine Reviews* 2(4):213–29.

Driver, J. S., D. J. Dijk, E. Werth, K. Biedermann, and A. Borbely. 1996. Sleep and the sleep electroencephalogram across the menstrual cycle in young healthy women. *Journal of Clinical Endocrinology and Metabolism* 81(2):728–35.

Durand, V. M., and J. A. Mindell. 1990. Behavioral treatment of multiple childhood sleep disorders. *Behavior Modification* 14:37–49.

———. 1993. Treatment of childhood sleep disorders: Generalization across disorders and effects on family members. *Journal of Pediatric Psychology* 18(6):731–50.

Duyff, R. 1996. *The American Dietetic Association's Complete Food and Nutrition Guide.* Minneapolis, Minn.: Chronimed Publishing.

Eastman, C. I., K. T. Stewart, M. P. Mahoney, L. Liu, and L. F. Fogg. 1994. Dark goggles and bright light improve circadian rhythm adaptation to night-shift work. *Sleep* 17:535–43.

Edinger, J. D., W. K. Wohlgemuth, R. A Radtke, G. R. Marsh, and R. E. Quillian. 2001. Cognitive behavioral therapy for treatment of chronic primary insomnia. *Journal of the American Medical Association* (JAMA) 28514:1856–1864.

Ehlers, C. L., and D. J. Kupfer. 1997. Slow-wave sleep: Do young adult men and women age differently? *Journal of Sleep Research* 6 (3):211–15.

Endometriosis Association 2000. *What is Endometriosis?* Endometriosis Association Web site http://www.endometriosisassn.org/endo.html.

Engleman, H. M., R. N. Kingshott, S. E. Martin, and N. J. Douglas. 2000. Cognitive function in the sleep apnea/hypopnea syndrome (SAHS). *Sleep* 23(Supplement 4):102–8.

Epsie, C. A., D. N. Brooks, and W. R. Lindsay. 1989. An evaluation of tailored psychological treatment of insomnia. *Journal of Behavior Therapy and Experimental Psychiatry* 20:143–54.

Epsie, C. A., W. R. Lindsay, D. N. Brooks, E. M. Hood, and T. Turvey. 1989. A controlled comparative investigation of psychological treatments for chronic sleep-onset insomnia. *Behaviour Research and Therapy* 27:79–88.

Evans, M. L., M. J. Dick, and A. S. Clark. 1995. Sleep during the week before labor: Relationships to labor outcomes. *Clinical Nursing Research* 4(3):238–52.

Ferber, R. 1985. *Solve Your Child's Sleep Problems.* New York: Simon and Schuster.

Fletcher, E. C. 2000. Hypertension in patients with sleep apnea, a combined effect? *Thorax* 55(9):726–28.

Ford, D. E., and D. B. Kamerow. 1989. Epidemiologic study of sleep disturbances and psychiatric disorders: An opportunity for prevention? *Journal of the American Medical Association* 262:1479–84.

France, K. G., J. M. T. Henderson, and S. M. Hudson. 1996. Fact, act, and tact: A three-stage approach to treating the sleep problems of infants and young children. In *Child and Adolescent Psychiatric Clinics of North America: Sleep Disorders*, edited by R. Dahl. Philadelphia: W. B. Saunders Company. 5(3):581–99.

Franco, P., J. Szliwowski, M. Dramaix, and A. Kahn. 1999. Decreased autonomic responses to obstructive sleep events in future victims of sudden infant death syndrome. *Pediatric Research* 46(1): 33–39.

Fryer, A. J., M. R. Liebowitz, J. M. Gorman, and R. Campeas. 1987. Discontinuation of alprazolam treatment in panic patients. *American Journal of Psychiatry* 144:303–308.

Futterman, A., L. Thompson, D. Gallagher-Thompson, and R. Ferris. 1995. Depression in late life: Epidemiology, assessment, etiology, and treatment. In *Handbook of Depression,* edited by E. E. Beckham and W. R. Leber. New York: Guilford Press.

Garey, A. I. 1999. *Weaving Work and Motherhood.* Philadelphia: Temple University Press.

George, C. F. 2000. Perspectives on the management of insomnia in patients with chronic respiratory disorders. *Sleep* 23(1)(Supplement):S31–35; discussion S36–38.

Goldenberg, D. L. 1993. Do infections trigger fibromyalgia? *Arthritis Rheumatology* 36:1489–92.

Goldenberg, D. L., D. T. Felson, and H. Dinerman. 1986. A randomized controlled trial of amitriptyline and naproxen in the treatment of patients with fibromyalgia. *Arthritis Rheumatology* 29:1371–77.

Goldmann, David R., and David A. Horowitz. 2000. *American College of Physicians Home Medical Guide to Migraine and Other Headaches.* New York: DK Publishing.

Goodman, J. D. S., C. Brodie, and G. A. Ayida. 1988. Restless legs syndrome in pregnancy. *British Medical Journal* 297:1101–2.

Greene, R. A., D. Lewis, E. T. Cabus, and O. A. Kletzky. 1995. Impaired sleep function associated with the menopause and the effects of estrogen replacement therapy. *American Society of Reproductive Medicine (ASRM) Abstracts.*

Guilleminault, C., and A. Anagnos. 2000. Narcolepsy. In *Principles and Practice of Sleep Medicine*, 3d ed., edited by M. H. Kryger, T. Roth, and W. C. Dement. Philadelphia: Saunders.

Guilleminault, C., M. Quera-Salva, M. Partinen, and A. Jamieson. 1988. Women and the obstructive sleep apnea syndrome. *Chest* 92:104–9.

Gupta, M. A., N. J. Schork, and C. Gay. 1992. Nocturnal leg cramps in pregnancy: A prospective study of clinical features. *Sleep Research* 21:294.

Hauri, P. J., M. Friedman, and C. L. Ravaris. 1989. Sleep in patients with spontaneous panic attacks. *Sleep* 12:323–37.

Hobson, J. A. 1989. *Sleep.* New York: Scientific American Library.

Hochschild, A. R. 1989. *The Second Shift.* New York: Avon.

Hoehn-Sarc, R., and D. R. McLeod. 1990. Generalized anxiety disorder in adulthood. In *Handbook of Child and Adult Psychopathology: A Longitudinal Perspective,* edited by M. Hersen and C. G. Last. New York: Pergamon Press.

Horne, J., and L. Reyner. 1999. Vehicle accidents related to sleep: A review. *Occupational and Environmental Medicine* 56:289–294.

Inamorato, E., S. N. Minatti-Hannuch, and E. Zukerman. 1993. The role of sleep in migraine attacks. *Arquivos de Neuro-psiquiatria* 51 (4):429–32.

International Food Information Council Foundation. 1998. *Everything You Need to Know about Caffeine.* International Food Information Council Foundation Web site http://ificinfo.health.org/brochure/caffeine.htm.

Jacobson, E. 1962. *You Must Relax.* New York: McGraw-Hill.

Jacobson, N. S., and S. D. Hollon. 1996. Cognitive-behavioral therapy versus pharmacotherapy: Now that the jury's returned its verdict, it's time to present the rest of the evidence. *Journal of Consulting and Clinical Psychology* 64:74–80.

Jacquinet-Salord, M. C., T. Lang, C. Fouriaud, I. Nicoulet, and A. Bingham. 1993. Sleeping tablet consumption, self reported quality of sleep, and working conditions. Group of Occupational Physicians of APSAT. *Journal of Epidemiological Community Health* 47(1):64–68.

Johnson, J. E. 1994. Sleep and alcohol use in rural old-old women. *Journal of Community Health Nursing* 11:211–218.

Johnson, J. E. 1997. Insomnia, alcohol, and over the counter drug use in old-old urban women. *Journal of Community Health Nursing* 14:181–188.

Karacan, I., W. Heine, H. W. Agnew, R. L. Williams, W. B. Webb, and J. J. Ross. 1968. Characteristics of sleep patterns during late pregnancy and the postpartum periods. *American Journal of Obstetrics and Gynecology* 101(5):579–85.

Keefe, D. L., R. Watson, and F. Naftolin. 1999. Hormone replacement therapy may alleviate sleep apnea in menopausal women: A pilot study. Menopause: *The Journal of the North American Menopause Society* 6(3):196–200.

Klosko, J. S., D. H. Barlow, R. Tassinari, and J. A. Cerny. 1990. A comparison of alprazolam and behavior therapy in treatment of panic disorder. *Journal of Consulting and Clinical Psychology* 58:77–84.

Koss, M. P., L. Heise, and N. P. Russo. 1994. The global health burden of rape. *Psychology of Women Quarterly* 18:509–537.

Kripke, D. F., M. R. Klauber, D. L. Wingard, R. L. Fell, J. D. Assmus, and L. Garfinkel. 1998. Mortality hazard associated with prescription hypnotics. *Biological Psychiatry* 43(9):687–93.

Krieger, J. 2000. Respiratory physiology: Breathing in normal subjects. In *Principles and Practice of Sleep Medicine*, 3d ed., edited by M. H. Kryger, T. Roth, and W. C. Dement. Philadelphia: Saunders.

Kronenberg, F. 1990. Hot flashes: Epidemiology and physiology. *Annals of the New York Academy of Science* 592:52–86; discussion 123–33.

Kryger, M. H. 2000. Management of obstructive sleep apnea-hypopnea syndrome: Overview. In *Principles and Practice of Sleep Medicine*, 3d ed., edited by M. H. Kryger, T. Roth, and W. C. Dement. Philadelphia: Saunders.

Kryger, M. H., T. Roth, and W. C. Dement. 2000. *Principles and Practice of Sleep Medicine*, 3d ed. Philadelphia: Saunders.

Kupfer, D. J., and F. G. Foster. 1972. Interval between onset of sleep and rapid-eye-movement sleep as an indicator of depression. *Lancet* 2:684–86.

Kupfer, D. J., and C. F. Reynolds III. 1983. Sleep disorders. *Hospital Practice* 18(2):101–5, 109–14, 117–19.

Kupfer, D. J., R. F. Ulrich, and P. A. Coble. 1985. Electroencephalographic sleep of younger depressives. *Archives of General Psychiatry* 42:806–10.

Lacks, P. 1987. *Behavioral Treatment for Persistent Insomnia.* New York: Pergamon Press.

Landrine, H. 1987. On the politics of madness: A preliminary analysis of the relationship between social roles and psychopathology. *Psychological Monographs* 113(3):341–406.

Lauersen, N., and C. DeSwann. 1988. *The Endometriosis Answer Book: New Hope, New Help.* New York: Rason Associates.

Laurence, L., and B. Weinhouse. 1994. *Outrageous Practices: The Alarming Truth about How Medicine Mistreats Women.* New York: Fawcett Columbine.

Lee, K. 1998. Alterations in sleep during pregnancy and postpartum. *Sleep Medicine Reviews* 2(4):231–42.

Lee, K. A. 1992. Self-reported sleep disturbances in employed women. *Sleep* 15:493–498.

Lee, K. A., G. McEnany, and M. E. Zaffke. 2000. REM sleep and mood state in childbearing women: Sleepy or weepy? *Sleep* 23 (7):877–84.

Lee, K. A., J. F. Shaver, E. C. Giblin, and N. F. Woods. 1990. Sleep patterns related to menstrual cycle phase and premenstrual affective symptoms. *Sleep* 13:403–9.

Lee, K. A., and D. L. Taylor. 1996. Is there a generic midlife woman? The health and symptom experience of midlife women. *Journal of the North American Menopause Society* 3:154–164.

Lewinsohn, P. M., H. Hoberman, L. Teri, and M. Hautziner. 1985. An integrative theory of depression. In *Theoretical Issues in Behavior Therapy*, edited by S. Reiss and R. Bootzin. Orlando, Fla.: Academic Press.

Lichstein, K. L., and B. W. Riedel. 1994. Behavioral assessment and treatment of insomnia: A review with an emphasis on clinical application. *Behavior Therapy* 25:659–88.

Lin, L., J. Faraco, R. Li, H. Kadotani, W. Rogers, X. Lin, X. Qiu, P. deJong, S. Nishino, and E. Mignot. 1999. The sleep disorder canine narcolepsy is caused by a mutation in the hypocretin (orexin) receptor 2 gene. *Cell* 98(3):365–76.

Lipton, R. B., W. F. Stewart, D. D. Celantano, and M. L. Reed. 1992. Undiagnosed migraine headaches: A comparison of symptom-based and reported physician diagnosis. *Archives of Internal Medicine* 152(6):1273–78.

Little, R. E., and J. K. Wendt. 1991. The effects of maternal drinking in the reproductive period: An epidemiologic review. *Journal of Substance Abuse* 3(2):187–204.

Loh, N. K., D. S. Dinner, N. Foldvary, F. Skobieranda, and W. W. Yew. 1999. Do patients with obstructive sleep apnea wake up with headaches? *Archives of Internal Medicine* 159(15):1765–68.

Loring, M., and B. Powell. 1988. Gender, race, and DSM-III: A study of the objectivity of psychiatric diagnostic behavior. *Journal of Health and Social Behavior* 29:1–22.

Love, S. 1997. What we really know about breast cancer and HRT. *Alternative Therapies in Health and Medicine* 3(5):82–90.

Lozoff, B. 1995. Culture and family: Influences on childhood sleep practices and problems. In *Principles and Practice of Sleep Medicine in the Child*, edited by R. Ferber and M. Kryger. Philadelphia: Saunders.

Lozoff, B., A. W. Wolf, and N. S. Davis. 1985. Sleep problems seen in pediatric practice. *Pediatrics* 183:477–83.

Lugaresi, E., S. Mondini, M. Zucconi, P. Montagna, and F. Cirignotta. 1983. Staging of heavy snorers' disease: A proposal. *Bulletin Europeen de Physiopathologie Respiratoire* 19(6):590–94.

Lugaresi, E., F. Cirginotta, M. Zucconi, S. Mondini, P. L. Lenzi, and G. Coccagna. 1983. Good and poor sleepers: An epidemiological survey of the San Marino population. In *Sleep/Wake Disorders: Natural History, Epidemiology, and Long-Term Evolution*, edited by C. Guilleminault and E. Lugaresi. New York: Raven Press.

Lydiard, R. B., O. Brawman-Mintzer, and J. C. Ballenger. 1996. Recent developments in the psychopharmacology of anxiety disorders. *Journal of Consulting and Clinical Psychology* 64:660–68.

Manber, R., and R. Bootzin. 1991. The effects of regular wake-up schedules on daytime sleepiness in college students. *Sleep Research* 20:284.

———. 1997. Sleep and the menstrual cycle. *Health Psychology* 16 (3):209–14.

Markowitz, J. C., and M. W. Weissman. 1995. Interpersonal psychotherapy. In *Handbook of Depression*, edited by E. E. Beckham and W. R. Leber. New York: Guilford Press.

Mauri, M. 1990. Sleep and the reproductive cycle: A review. *Health Care for Women International* 11(4):409–21.

McCain, G. A., D. A. Bell, F. M. Mai, and P. D. Halliday. 1988. A controlled study of the effects of a supervised cardiovascular fitness training program on the manifestations of primary fibromyalgia. *Arthritis Rheumatology* 31(9):1135–41.

McKenna, J, E. Thomas, T. Anders, A. Sadeh, V. Schechtman, and S. Glotzbach. 1993. Infant-parent co-sleeping in an evolutionary perspective: Implications for understanding infant sleep development and the sudden death syndrome. *Sleep* 16:263–82.

Mellman, T. A., and T. W. Uhde. 1989. Sleep panic attacks: New clinical findings and theoretical implications. *American Journal of Psychiatry* 146:1204–7.

Mignot, E. 2000. Pathophysiology of narcolepsy. In *Principles and Practice of Sleep Medicine*, 3d ed., edited by M. H. Kryger, T. Roth, and W. C. Dement. Philadelphia: Saunders.

Mindell, J. A., and B. J. Jacobson. 1997. Sleep disturbances across pregnancy: A pilot study. *Sleep Research* 26:572.

————. 2000. Sleep disturbances during pregnancy. *Journal of Obstetric, Gynecologic, and Neonatal Nursing* 29(6):590–97.

Mitler, M., W. C. Dement, and D. F. Dinges. 2000. Sleep medicine, public policy, and public health. In *Principles and Practice of Sleep Medicine* edited by M. H. Kryger, T. Roth, and W. C. Dement. Philadelphia, Pa.: Saunders.

Moe, K. E. 1999. Reproductive hormones, aging, and sleep. *Seminars in Reproductive Endocrinology* 17(4):339–48.

Moldofsky, H. 1995. Sleep, neuroimmine and neuroendocrine functions in fibromyalgia and chronic fatigue syndrome. *Advances in Neuroimmunology* 5:39–56.

Moldofsky, H., P. Scarisbrick, R. England, and H. A. Smythe. 1975. Musculoskeletal symptoms and nonREM sleep disturbance in patients with "fibrositis syndrome" and healthy subjects. *Psychosomatic Medicine* 34:341–51.

Monk, T. H., and J. A. Wagner. 1989. Social factors can outweigh biological ones in determining night shift safety. *Human Factors* 31:721–24.

Moore, R. Y., and V. B. Eichler. 1972. Loss of a circadian adrenal corticosterone rhythm following suprachiasmatic lesions in the rat. *Brain Research* 42:201–206.

Moore-Ede, M. 1998. *Working Nights Health & Safety Guide.* Cambridge: Circadian Information.

Montplaisir, J., A. Nicolas, R. Godbout, and A. Walters. 2000. Restless legs syndrome and periodic limb movement disorders. In *Principles and Practice of Sleep Medicine,* 3d ed., edited by M. H. Kryger, T. Roth, and W. C. Dement. Philadelphia: Saunders.

Morin, C. M. 1993. *Insomnia: Psychological Assessment and Management.* New York: Guilford Press.

Morin, C. M., C. A. Colecchi, J. Stone, R. Sood, and D. Brink. 1995. Cognitive behavior therapy and pharmacotherapy for insomnia: Update of a placebo-controlled clinical trial. *Sleep Research* 24:303.

Morin, C. M., J. P. Culbert, and S. M. Schwartz. 1994. Nonpharmacological interventions for insomnia: A meta-analysis of treatment efficacy. *American Journal of Psychiatry* 151:1172–80.

Mortola, J. F. 1994. A risk-benefit appraisal of drugs used in the management of premenstrual syndrome. *Drug Safety* 10(2):160–69.

National Fibromyalgia Parnership, Inc. 1999. An overview of the fundamental features of fibromyalgia syndrome. *FMS Monograph* Web site http://www.fmpartnership.org/FMPartnership.htm.

National Institutes of Health. 1991. *Women's Health Initiative.* Bethesda, Md.: National Institutes of Health, Office for Research on Women's Health.

National Institute of Mental Health. 1999. *The Invisible Disease: Depression.* Bethesda, Md.: National Institute of Mental Health, Information Resources and Inquiries Branch.

National Institute for Occupational Safety and Health. 1997. *Plain Language About Shiftwork.* Washington, D.C.: National Institute for Occupational Safety and Health.

National Sleep Foundation. 1998. *Women and Sleep Poll.* Washington, D.C.: National Sleep Foundation.

———. 2000. *Treating Insomnia in the Primary Care Setting.* Washington, D.C.: National Sleep Foundation.

———. 2000. *Sleep in America Poll.* Washington, D.C.: National Sleep Foundation.

Nolen-Hoeksema, S. 1990. *Sex Differences in Depression.* Stanford, Calif.: Stanford University Press.

———. 1995. Gender differences in coping with depression across the lifespan. *Depression* 3:81–90.

———. 1998. *Abnormal Psychology.* Boston: McGraw-Hill.

O'Hara, M. W. 1987. Postpartum "blues," depression, and psychosis: A review. *Journal of Psychosomatic Obstetrics and Gynecology* 7:205–227.

Orr, W. C. 1997. Obstructive sleep apnea: Natural history and varieties of the clinical presentation. In *Understanding Sleep: The Evaluation and Treatment of Sleep Disorders,* edited by M. R. Pressman and W. C. Orr. Washington, D.C.: American Psychological Association.

Owens, J. F., and K. A. Mathews. 1998. Sleep disturbance in healthy middle-aged women. *Maturitas: The European Menopause Journal* 30:41–50.

Paret, I. 1983. Night waking and its relation to mother-infant interaction in nine-month-old infants. In *Frontiers of Infant Psychiatry,* edited by J. Call, E. Galenson, and R. L. Tyson. New York: Basic Books.

Parlee, M. B. 1994. Commentary on the literature review. In *Premenstrual Dysphorias,* edited by J. H. Gold and S. K. Severino. Washington, D.C.: American Psychiatric Association.

Phillips, B. A., and F. J. Danner. 1995. Cigarette smoking and sleep disturbance. *Archives of Internal Medicine* 155:734–737.

Pilcher, J. J., and A. I. Huffcutt. 1996. Effects of sleep deprivation on performance: A meta-analysis. *Sleep* 194:318–26.

Pillitteri, J. L., L. T. Kozlowski, D. C. Person, and M. E. Spear. 1994. Over-the-counter sleep aids: Widely used but rarely studied. *Journal of Substance Abuse* 6:315–23.

Quillen, S. I. M. 1997. Infant and mother sleep patterns during fourth postpartum week. *Comprehensive Pediatric Nursing* 20:115–23.

Rains, J., and F. Sheftell, eds. 2000. *Women and Migraine.* American Council for Headache Education Web site http://www. achenet.org/women.

Roehrs, T. 1993. Caffeine. In *Encyclopedia of Sleep and Dreaming,* edited by M. A. Carskadon, A. Rechtschaffen, G. Firchardson, T. Roth, and J. M. Siegel. New York: Macmillan.

Roehrs, T., and T. Roth. 1997. Hypnotics, alcohol, and caffeine: Relation to insomnia. In *Understanding Sleep: The Evaluation and Treatment of Sleep Disorders,* edited by M. R. Pressman and W. C. Orr. Washington, D.C.: American Psychological Association.

———. 2000. Hypnotics: Efficacy and adverse effects. In *Principles and Practice of Sleep Medicine,* edited by M. H. Kryger, T. Roth, and W. C. Dement. Philadelphia: Saunders.

Roehrs, T., F. Zorick, and T. Roth. 2000. Transient and short-term insomnia. In *Principles and Practice of Sleep Medicine,* edited by M. H. Kryger, T. Roth, and W. C. Dement. Philadelphia: Saunders.

Rollins, J. H. 1996. *Women's Minds, Women's Bodies: The Psychology of Women in a Biosocial Context.* Upper Saddle River, N.J.: Prentice-Hall, Inc.

Rothenberg, S. A. 1997. Introduction to sleep disorders. In *Understanding Sleep: the Evaluation and Treatment of Sleep Disorders,* edited by M. R. Pressman and W. C. Orr. Washington, D.C.: American Psychological Association.

Salzarulo, P. 1987. Long lasting disturbances in women after childbirth. *Journal of Reproductive and Infant Psychology* 5:245–46.

Saskin, P. 1997. Obstructive sleep apnea: Treatment options, efficacy, and effects. In *Understanding Sleep: the Evaluation and Treatment of Sleep Disorders,* edited by M. R. Pressman and W. C. Orr. Washington, D.C.: American Psychological Association.

Sateia, M. J., K. Doghramji, P. J. Hauri, and C. M. Morin. 2000. Evaluation of chronic insomnia: An American Academy of Sleep Medicine review. *Sleep* 223(2):243–308.

Saurel-Cubizolles, M.J., P. Romito, N. Lelong, and P. Y. Ancel. 2000. Women's health after childbirth: A longitudinal study in France and Italy. *British Journal of Obstetrics and Gynecology* 107(10): 1202–9.

Schmidt-Nowara, W. W., D. B. Coultas, C. Wiggins, B. E. Skipper, and J. M. Samet. 1990. Snoring in a Hispanic-American population: Risk factors and association with hypertension and other morbidity. *Archives of Internal Medicine* 150(3):597–601.

Schmidt-Nowara, W. W, T. E. Meade, and M. B. Hays. 1991. Treatment of snoring and obstructive sleep apnea with a dental orthosis. *Chest* 99:1378–85.

Scott, G., and M. P. M. Richards. 1990. Nightwaking in one-year-old children in England. *Child: Care, Health, and Development* 16:283–302.

Shader, R. I., D. J. Greenblatt, and M. B. Balter. 1991. Appropriate use and regulatory control of benzodiazepines. *Journal of Clinical Pharmacology* 31(9):781–84.

Shaver, J., E. Giblin, M. Lentz, and K. Lee. 1988. Sleep patterns and stability in perimenopausal women. *Sleep* 11(6):556–61.

Shapiro, C. M., and W. C. Dement. 1994. ABC of sleep disorders: Impact and epidemiology of sleep disorders. *British Medical Journal* 306:1604–7.

Simon, J. A., J. Hsia, J. A. Cauley, C. Richards, F. Harris, J. Fong, E. Barrett-Connor, and S. B. Hulley. 2001. Postmenopausal hormone therapy and risk of stroke: The heart and estrogen-progestin replacement study. *Circulation* 103(5):638–42.

Smolensky, M., and L. Lamberg. 2000. *The Body Clock Guide to Better Health.* New York: Henry Holt and Company.

Spielman A. J., P. Saskin, and M. J. Thorpy. 1987. Treatment of chronic insomnia by restriction of time in bed. *Sleep* 10(1):45–56.

Spielman, A. J., and P. B. Glovinsky. 1997. The diagnostic interview and differential diagnosis for complaints of insomnia. In *Understanding Sleep: The Evaluation and Treatment of Sleep Disorders,* edited by M. R. Pressman and W. C. Orr. Washington, D.C.: American Psychological Association.

St. Amand, R. P., and C. C. Marek. 1999. *What Your Doctor May Not Tell You About Fibromyalgia.* New York: Warner Books.

Steinberg, K. K., S. B. Thacker, S. J. Smith, D. F. Stroup, M. M. Zack, W. D. Flanders, and R. L. Berkelman. 1991. A meta-analysis of the effect of estrogen replacement therapy on the risk of breast cancer. *Journal of the American Medical Association* 265(15): 1985–90.

Stewart, W. F., R. B. Lipton, E. Chee, J. Sawyer, and S. D. Silberstein. 2000. Menstrual cycle and headache in a population sample of migraineurs. *Neurology* 55(10):17–23.

Stewart, W. F., R. B. Lipton, J. Whyte, A. Dowson, K. Kolodner, J. N. Liberman, and J. Sawyer. 1999. An international study to assess reliability of the Migraine Disability Assessment (MIDAS) score. *Neurology* 53(5):988–94.

Strickland, B. R. 1992. Women and depression. *Current Directions in Psychological Science* 1(4):132–35.

Sullivan, C. E., M. Berthon-Jones, F. G. Issa, and L. Evers. 1981. Reversal of obstructive sleep apnea by continuous positive airway pressure applied through the nares. *Lancet* 1:862–65.

Tanz, R. R., and J. Charrow. 1993. Black clouds: Work load, sleep, and resident reputation. *American Journal of Diseases of Children* 147:579–84.

Telch, M. J., J. A. Lucas, and P. Nelson. 1989. Nonclinical panic in college students: An investigation of prevalence and symptomatology. *Journal of Abnormal Psychology* 98:300–6.

Tribotti, S., N. Lyons, S. Blackburn, M. Stein, and J. Withers. 1988. Nursing diagnoses for the postpartum woman. *Journal of Obstetric, Gynecologic, and Neonatal Nursing* 17(6):410–16.

Uhde, T. W. 2000. Anxiety disorders. In *Principles and Practice of Sleep Medicine*, edited by M. H. Kryger, T. Roth, and W. C. Dement. Philadelphia: Saunders.

Ulfberg, J., N. Carter, M. Talback, and C. Edling. 2000. Adverse health effects among women living with heavy snorers. *Health Care for Women International* 21(2):81–90.

Unger, R., and M. Crawford. 1992. *Women and Gender: A Feminist Psychology.* New York: McGraw-Hill.

Urponen, H., I. Vuori, J. Hasan, and M. Partinen. 1988. Self-evaluations of factors promoting and disturbing sleep: An epidemiological survey in Finland. *Social Science and Medicine* 26 (4):443–50.

U.S. Bureau of the Census. 1999. *Statistical Abstract of the United States.* 1999. Washington, D.C.: U.S. Bureau of the Census.

U.S. Department of Labor, Women's Bureau. 1994. *Working Women Count Survey.* Washington, D.C.: U.S. Department of Labor, Women's Bureau.

———. 1994. *Report to the Nation, Executive Summary.* Washington, D.C.: U.S. Department of Labor, Women's Bureau.

————. 1999. *Twenty Facts on Women Workers.* U.S. Department of Labor, Women's Bureau Web site http://www.dol.gov/dol/wb/public/wb_pubs/20fact00.htm.

————. 2000. *Twenty Facts on Women Workers.* U.S. Department of Labor, Women's Bureau Web site http://www.dol.gov/dol/wb/public/wb_pubs/20fact00.htm.

Utley, M. J. 1995. *Narcolepsy: A funny disorder that's no laughing matter.* DeSoto, Tex.: M. J. Utley.

Van Tassel, E. B. 1985. The relative influence of child and environmental characteristics on sleep disturbances in the first and second years of life. *Developmental and Behavioral Pediatrics* 6(2): 81–86.

Verbrugge, L. M. 1983. Multiple roles and physical health of women and men. *Journal of Health and Social Behavior* 24(1):16–30.

Vitiello, M. V. 1997. Sleep disorders and aging: Understanding the causes. *The Journals of Gerontology. Series A, Biological Sciences and Medical Sciences* 52(4):189–91.

Walker, L, and Best. 1991. Well being of mothers with infant children: A preliminary comparison of employed women and homemakers. *Women and Health* 17(1):71–89.

Warr, P., and G. Parry. 1982. Paid employment and women's psychological well-being. *Psychological Bulletin* 91:498–516.

Waters, M. A., and K. A. Lee. 1996. Differences between primigravidae and multigravidae mothers in sleep disturbances, fatigue, and functional status. *Journal of Nurse-Midwifery.* 41(5): 364–67.

Webb, W. B. 1985. A further analysis of age and sleep deprivation effects. *Psychophysiology* 22(2):156–61.

————. 1992. *Sleep: The Gentle Tyrant.* 2d ed. Bolton, Mass.: Anker Publishing Company.

Wehr, T. A. 1991. The durations of human melatonin secretion and sleep respond to changes in daylength (photoperiod). *Journal of Clinical Endocrinology and Metabolism* 73(6):1276–80.

Weissbluth, M. 1987. *Healthy Sleep Habits, Happy Children.* New York: Fawcett Columbine.

Wilkie, C., and C. M. Shapiro. 1992. Sleep deprivation and the postnatal blues. *Journal of Psychosomatic Research* 36(4):309–16.

Wolfe, F. 1993. The epidemiology of fibromyalgia. *Journal of Musculoskeletal Pain* 1(3/4):137–48.

Wolfe, F., D. J. Hawley, M. A. Cathey, X. Caro, and I. J. Russell. 1985. Fibrositis: Symptom frequency and criteria for diagnosis. An evaluation of 291 rheumatic disease patients and 58 normal individuals. *Journal of Rheumatology* 12:1159–63.

Wolfson, A. R., and U. Anwer. 2000. *Sleep and Affect in Pregnancy and Postpartum Months.* Paper presented at the Annual Meeting of the Northeast Sleep Society, Worcester, Mass.

Wolfson, A. R., and M. A. Carskadon. 1998. Sleep schedules and daytime functioning in adolescents. *Child Development* 69(4):875–87.

Wolfson, A. R., P. Lacks, and A. Futterman. 1992. Effects of parent training on infant sleeping patterns, parents' stress, and perceived parental competence. *Journal of Consulting and Clinical Psychology* 60(1):41–48.

Wood, C., and D. Jakubowicz. 1980. The treatment of premenstrual symptoms with mefenamic acid. *British Journal of Obstetrics and Gynaecology* 87(7):627–30.

Woodward, S., and R. R. Freedman. 1994. The thermoregulatory effects of menopausal hot flashes on sleep. *Sleep* 17(6):497–501.

Young, T., J. Blustein, L. Finn, and M. Palta. 1997. Sleep-disordered breathing and motor vehicle accidents in a population-based sample of employed adults. *Sleep* 208:608–613

Young, T., L. Evans, L. Finn, and M. Palta. 1997. Estimation of the clinically diagnosed proportion of sleep apnea syndrome in middle-aged men and women. *Sleep* 20(9):705–6.

Young, T., M. Palta, J. Dempsey, J. Skatrud, S. Weber, and S. Badr. 1993. The occurrence of sleep-disordered breathing among middle-aged adults. *New England Journal of Medicine* 328 (17):1230–35.

Young, T., and P. Peppard. 2000. Sleep-disordered breathing and cardiovascular disease: Epidemiologic evidence for a relationship. *Sleep* 23(Supplement)(4):S122–26.

Zammit, G. K. 1997. Delayed sleep phase syndrome and related conditions. In *Understanding Sleep: The Evaluation and Treatment of Sleep Disorders,* edited by M. R. Pressman and W. C. Orr. Washington, D.C.: American Psychological Association.

Zuckerman, B., J. Stevenson, and V. Bailey. 1987. Sleep problems in early childhood: Continuities, predictive factors, and behavioral correlates. *Pediatrics* 80:664–71.

Index

Some Other New Harbinger Titles

Watercooler Wisdom, Item 4364 $14.95

The Juicy Tomato Guide to Ripe Living After 50, Item 4321 $16.95

What's Right With Me, Item 4429 $16.95

The Balanced Mom, Item 4534 $14.95

Women Who Worry Too Much, Item 4127 $13.95

In Harm's Way, Item 4003 $14.95

Breastfeeding Made Simple, Item 4046 $16.95

The Well-Ordered Office, Item 3856 $13.95

Talk to Me, Item 3317 $12.95

Romantic Intelligence, Item 3309 $15.95

Transformational Divorce, Item 3414 $13.95

The Rape Recovery Handbook, Item 3376 $15.95

Eating Mindfully, Item 3503 $13.95

Sex Talk, Item 2868 $12.95

Everyday Adventures for the Soul, Item 2981 $11.95

A Woman's Addiction Workbook, Item 2973 $19.95

The Daughter-In-Law's Survival Guide, Item 2817 $12.95

PMDD, Item 2833 $13.95

The Vulvodynia Survival Guide, Item 2914 $16.95

Love Tune-Ups, Item 2744 $10.95

Brave New You, Item 2590 $13.95

The Woman's Book of Sleep, Item 2418 $14.95

Pregnancy Stories, Item 2361 $14.95

The Women's Guide to Total Self-Esteem, Item 2418 $14.95

The Conscious Bride, Item 2132 $12.95

Call **toll free, 1-800-748-6273,** or log on to our online bookstore at **www.newharbinger.com** to order. Have your Visa or Mastercard number ready. Or send a check for the titles you want to New Harbinger Publications, Inc., 5674 Shattuck Ave., Oakland, CA 94609. Include $4.50 for the first book and 75¢ for each additional book, to cover shipping and handling. (California residents please include appropriate sales tax.) Allow two to five weeks for delivery.

Prices subject to change without notice.